English-Spanish Terms in

SPEECH, LANGUAGE, AND HEARING

2nd Edition

With translations for SLPs, audiologists, interpreters, and more

Con traducciones para fonoaudiólogos, audiólogos, intérpretes y más

Contents

Guide to the English-Spanish Terms

This book offers a comprehensive list of terms that are common to the studies of speech, language, and hearing, most notably speech-language pathology, but also including terms relevant to audiology, linguistics, neurology and pedagogy. It should be said that no single reference can truly capture the wide breadth of terminology and jargon that exists in these domains. Nonetheless, this book attempts to cover the most important word selections that are relevant to many different types of SLPs and other professionals in a variety of settings. The purpose of this book is to serve as a translation reference, aiding in the development of bilingual skills relevant to the field and bridging the gap between SLPs of different backgrounds.

Names and abbreviations of standardized assessments, such as the CLQT+, are not included in this glossary or its appendices. However, many widely used procedures, which are not considered standardized assessments, are named in this book.

English words and phrases are listed in alphabetical order based on the first letter of the word or the first word in the phrase. The translations in Spanish are not alphabetized for this section since they are correlated to the English terms.

All significant words in both English and Spanish entries are capitalized for consistency.

The English word or phrase being translated is printed in **bold.**

The word or phrase is followed by an *italicized* letter indicating the part of speech of the translation. For the Spanish translations, noun gender is represented by *f.* (feminine) or *m.* (masculine). Other abbreviations for part of speech include *a.* (adjective) and *v.* (verb). Some nouns, especially those representing people, can be masculine or feminine and are thus denoted by *m/f.* When a word is plural in the translation given, a *p.* will follow the part of speech.

The Spanish translation of the word follows the part of speech and is printed in plain text.

Spanish adjectives that change endings depending on the noun's gender are represented first by the masculine form, then by the alternative feminine ending, led by a hyphen (Subglótico-a). Spanish nouns that change endings with gender are represented the same way.

Both English verbs and their Spanish translations are presented in the infinitive form of the verb, except when a specific term is nearly always found in a different form.

Phrases that have common abbreviations will indicate that abbreviation in parentheses at the end of the phrase. The translated phrase will also include the abbreviation most used in the opposite language. In some cases, the abbreviation may be different for the translation, while other times, the Spanish abbreviation may be the same as the English one despite the Spanish translation having different letters or letter order. In these cases, the Spanish translation usually still uses the English abbreviation. See Appendix I to quickly reference a list of selected abbreviations in English, or Appendix II for abbreviations in Spanish.

When an entry has more than one common translation, the translations are separated by semicolons. Each new translation will be preceded by its own part of speech. The preferred or most widely used translation will appear first, followed by its other possible variations.

Some words may appear multiple times in different contexts or as part of other phrases. Other words may appear in different forms or different parts of speech as separate entries, when the difference between the two is significant in translation or when both versions are used frequently. Some nouns and adjectives may appear as separate entries as well as in a combined phrase, when appropriate.

The section that follows is the collection of English-Spanish translations. For the Spanish-English terms, see page 163.

A

Abdomen *m.* Abdomen

Abdominal *a.* Abdominal

Abducens Nerve *m.* Nervio Abducens; *m.* Nervio Motor Ocular Externo (MOT); *m.* Nervio Abducente

Abduct *v.* Abducir

Abduction *f.* Abducción

Abduction Quotient *m.* Cociente de Abducción

Ablation *f.* Ablación

Ableism *f.* Discriminación por las Discapacidades

Abnormality *f.* Anormalidad; *f.* Anomalía

Aboulia *f.* Abulia

Abstraction *f.* Abstracción

Abuse *m.* Abuso

Acalculia *f.* Acalculia

Accent *m.* Acento

Accent Mark *f.* Tilde ; *m.* Acento Ortográfico

Access Barriers *f.p.* Barreras de Acceso

Accessibility *f.* Accesibilidad

Accessory Nerve *m.* Nervio Accesorio; *m.* Nervio Espinal Accessorio

Accredited *a.* Acreditado-a

Acculturation *f.* Aculturación

Accuracy *f.* Exactitud

Achalasia *f.* Acalasia

Acoustic *a.* Acústico-a

Acoustic Nerve *m.* Nervio Coclear

Acoustic Neuroma *f.* Neurinoma del Acústico; *f.* Neurinoma Vestibular; *f.* Schwanoma Vestibular

Acquired Brain Injury (ABI) *f.* Lesión Cerebral Adquirida (LCA)

Acquired Immunodeficiency Syndrome (AIDS) *m.* Síndrome de Inmunodeficiencia Adquirida

Acquired Speech Disorder *m.* Trastorno Adquirido del Habla

Acquisition *f.* Adquisición

Action Potential *m.* Potencial de Acción

Activities of Daily Living (ADL) *f.p* Actividades de la Vida Diaria (ACVD)

Acute *a.* Agudo-a; *a.* Grave

Acute Care *f.* Atención de Agudos; *m.* Cuidado Intensivo

Adam's Apple *f.* Nuez de Adán; *f.* Manzana de Adán

Adaptation *f.* Adaptación

Adduct *v.* Aducir

Adduction *f.* Aducción

Adolescent *a.* Adolescente

Adult *a.* Adulto-a

Advocacy *f.* Defensa

Advocate *v.* Abogar

Aerodigestive *a.* Aerodigestivo-a

Afferent *a.* Aferente

Affix *m.* Afijo

Affricate *f.* Africada; *a.* Africado-a

African-American Vernacular English (AAVE) *m.* Inglés Afroestadounidense Vernáculo (IAV)

Ageism *m.* Edadismo; *m.* Viejismo; *f.* Discriminación por Edad

Aging *m.* Envejecimiento

Agnosia *f.* Agnosia

Agrammatic PPA *f.* APP Agramática; *f.* APP No Fluente

Agrammatism *m.* Agramatismo

Agraphia *f.* Agrafia

Aided Communication *f.* Comunicación Asistida

Air-Bone Gap *m.* Intervalo Aéreo-Óseo

Air Conduction *f.* Conducción Aérea

Air Pressure *f.* Presión de Aire

Airflow *m.* Flujo de Aire

Airway *f.p* Vías Respiratorias

Akinesia *f.* Acinesia

[13]

Akinetic *a.* Acinético-a

Alalia *f.* Alalia

Alexia *f.* Alexia

Allergic *a.* Alérgico-a

Allergy *f.* Alergia

Allophone *m.* Alófono

Alphabet *m.* Alfabeto; *m.* Abecedario

Alphabet Supplementation *f.* Suplementación del Alfabeto

Altered Speech *f.* Habla Modificada

Alveolar *a.* Alveolar

Alveolar Process *m.* Proceso Alveolar

Alveolar Ridge *f.* Cresta Alveolar; *m.p.* Alvéolos

Alveoli *m.p.* Alvéolos

Alveopalatal *a.* Alveopalatal

Alzheimer's Disease *f.* Enfermedad de Alzheimer

American Sign Language (ASL) *f.* Lengua de Signos Americana (ASL)

[14]

American Speech-Language-Hearing Association (ASHA) *f.* Asociación Americana del Habla, Lenguaje y Audición (ASHA)

Americans with Disabilities Act (ADA) *f.* Ley Sobre Estadounidenses con Discapacidades (ADA)

Amnesia *f.* Amnesia

Amplification *f.* Amplificación

Amplitude *f* Amplitud

Amyotrophic Lateral Sclerosis (ALS) *f.* Esclerosis Lateral Amiotrófica (ELA)

Analysis *m.* Análisis

Anaphylaxis *f.* Anafilaxia

Anarthria *f.* Anartria

Anastomosis *f.* Anastomosis

Anatomy *f.* Anatomía

Anencephaly *f.* Anencefalia

Anesthesia *f.* Anestesia

Anesthesiologist *m/f.* Anestesiólogo-a

Aneurism *m.* Aneurisma

Angiography *f.* Angiografía

Angular Gyrus *m.* Giro Angular

Ankyloglossia *f.* Anquiloglosia

Annual Review *f.* Revisión Anual

Anomia *f.* Anomia

Anomic Aphasia *f.* Afasia Anómica

Anopsia *f.* Anopsia

Anorexia *f.* Anorexia

Anotia *f.* Anotia

Anoxia *f.* Anoxia

Anterior *a.* Anterior

Anterior Cerebral Artery (ACA) *f.* Arteria Cerebral Anterior (ACA)

Anterior Commissure *f.* Comisura Anterior

Anterior Horn (Spinal Cord) *m.* Cuerno Anterior (de la Médula Espinal)

Anterograde Amnesia (AA) *f.* Amnesia Anterógrada (AA)

Anthropology *f.* Antropología

Aorta *f.* Aorta

Aperture *f.* Abertura

Apex *m.* Ápice

Apgar Score *f.* Puntuación de Apgar

Aphasia *f.* Afasia

Aphasic *a.* Afásico-a

Aphonia *f.* Afonía

Apical *a.* Apical

Apoplexy *f.* Apoplejía; *m.* Ictus

Apoptosis *f.* Apoptosis

Appendicular *a.* Apendicular

Applied Behavior Analysis (ABA) *m.* Análisis del Comportamiento Aplicado (ABA)

Applied Linguistics *f.* Lingüística Aplicada

Approach *m.* Enfoque; *m.* Planteamiento

Approximant *f.* Aproximante; *a.* Aproximante

Apraxia *f.* Apraxia

Apraxia of Speech (AOS) *f.* Apraxia del Habla (AOS)

Aprosodia *f.* Aprosodia

Aptitude *f.* Aptitud

Arachnoid Mater *f.* Aracnoides

Arcuate Fasciculus *m.* Fascículo Arqueado

Arteriovenous Malformation (AVM) *f.* Malformación Arteriovenosa (MAV)

Artery *f.* Arteria

Arthritis *f.* Artritis

Articulation *f.* Articulación

Articulators *m.* Articuladores

Articulatory Groping *f.* Articulación con Tanteo; *f.* Articulación a Tientas

Articulatory Phonetics *f.* Fonética Articulatoria

Aryepiglottal *a.* Ariepiglotal

Aryepiglottic Folds *m.p* Pliegues Ariepiglóticos

Arytenoid Adduction *f.* Aducción Aritenoidea

Arytenoids *f.* Aritenoides

Asemia *f.* Asemia

Asperger Syndrome (AS) *m.* Síndrome de Asperger (AS)

Asphyxiation *f.* Asfixia

Aspirate *v.* Aspirar

Aspirated *a.* Aspirado-a

Aspiration *f.* Aspiración

Aspiration Pneumonia *f.* Neumonía por Aspiración

Aspiration Pneumonitis *f.* Neumonitis por Aspiración

Assessment *f.* Evaluación

Assibilation *f.* Asibilación; *m.* Rehilamiento

Assimilation *f.* Asimilación

Asthma *f.* Asma

Asthmatic *a.* Asmático-a

Astrocyte *m.* Astrocito

[19]

Asymmetrical *a.* Asimétrico -a

Asymmetry *f.* Asimetría

Asymptomatic *a.* Asintomático-a

Ataxia *f.* Ataxia

Ataxic *a.* Atáxico-a

Ataxic Dysarthria *f.* Disartria Atáxica

Athetosis *f.* Atetosis

Atresia *f.* Atresia

Atrophy *f.* Atrofia

Attention Deficit Hyperactivity Disorder (ADHD) *m.* Trastorno por Déficit de Atención con Hiperactividad (TDAH)

Attention Span *m.* Periodo de Atención; *f.* Capacidad de Atención

Attenuation *f.* Atenuación

Attested *a.* Atestiguado-a

Audiogram *m.* Audiograma

Audiologist *m.* Audiólogo

Audiology *f.* Audiología

Audiometer *m.* Audiómetro

Audiometry *f.* Audiometría

Audition *f.* Audición

Auditory Brainstem Implant (ABI) *m.* Implante Auditivo de Tronco Cerebral (IATC)

Auditory Brainstem Response (ABR) *f.* Respuesta Auditiva del Tronco Encefálico (RATE)

Auditory Comprehension *f.* Comprensión Auditiva

Auditory Nerve *m.* Nervio Coclear

Auditory Verbal Agnosia (AVA) *f.* Sordera Verbal

Auditory-Verbal Therapy (AVT) *f.* Terapia Auditivo-Verbal (TAV)

Augmentation *m.* Aumento

Augmentative and Alternative Communication (AAC) *f.* Comunicación Aumentativa y Alternativa (CAA); *f.* Sistemas Aumentativos y Alternativos de Comunicación (SAAC)

Aural Rehabilitation *f.* Rehabilitación Auditiva

[21]

Auricle *m.* Pabellón Auricular

Auscultation *f.* Auscultación

Autism *m.* Autismo

Autism Spectrum Disorder (ASD) *m.* Trastornos del Espectro del Autismo (TEA)

Autoimmune Disease *f.* Enfermedad Autoinmunitaria

Autonomic Nervous System *m.* Sistema Nervioso Autónomo

Autopsy *f.* Autopsia

Axial *a.* Axial

Axis *m.* Eje

Axon *m.* Axón

B

Babble *v.* Balbucear

Babbling *m.* Balbuceo

Babinski's Sign *m.* Síntoma de Babinski

Baby Talk *m.* Lenguaje de Bebé; *m.* Maternés

Back Vowel *f.* Vocal Posterior

Backed *a.* Retraído-a; *a.* Posteriorizado-a

Backflow *m.* Reflujo

Backing *f.* Posteriorización; *f.* Retracción

Barium *m.* Bario

Barium Swallow *f.* Esofagografía con Bario; *f.* Deglución de Bario

Basal Ganglia *m.p.* Ganglios Basales

Base *f.* Base

Baseline *f.* Base; *f.* Referencia

Basilar Artery *f.* Arteria Basilar

Basilar Membrane *f.* Membrana Basilar

[23]

Bedside Examination *m.* Examen al Lado del Paciente

Bedside Manner *m.p.* Modales; *m.* Trato

Behavior *m.* Comportamiento; *f.* Conducta

Behind the Ear Hearing Aid (BTE) *m.* Audífono Retroauricular (BTE); *m.* Audífono Detrás de la Oreja (BTE)

Bell's Palsy *f.* Parálisis de Bell

Benign *a.* Benigno-a

Bias *m.* Sesgo; *f.* Parcialidad; *m.* Prejuicio

Bilabial *a.* Bilabial

Bilateral *a.* Bilateral

Bilateral Vocal Cord Paralysis *f.* Parálisis Bilateral de las Cuerdas Vocales

Bilingual *a.* Bilingüe

Bilirubin *f.* Bilirrubina

Binaural *a.* Binaural

Biopsy *f.* Biopsia

Bipolar Disorder *m.* Trastorno Bipolar

Bite *f.* Mordida; *f.* Oclusión

Bite Block *f.* Pieza de Mordida; *m.* Bloque de Mordida

Blend *m.* Grupo Consonántico; *f.* Combinación Consonántica

Blindness *f.* Ceguera

Blissymbols *m.p* Símbolos Bliss

Blocking *f.* Obstrucción; *f.* Interrupción

Blood-Brain Barrier (BBB) *f.* Barrera Hematoencefálica (BHE)

Board Certified Behavior Analyst (BCBA) *m/f.* Analista del Comportamiento Acreditado-a (BCBA)

Body Awareness *f.* Conciencia Corporal

Bolus *m.* Bolo; Bolus

Bone-Anchored Hearing Aid (BAHA) *m.* Audífono con Anclaje Óseo (BAHA); *m.* Implante Auditivo Osteointegrado (AOI); *m.* Audífono/Implante Anclado al Hueso (BAHA); *m.* Audífono de Conducción Ósea (BAHA)

Bone Conduction *f.* Conducción Ósea

Bony Labyrinth *m.* Laberinto Óseo

Borderline Personality Disorder (BPD) *m.* Trastorno Límite de la Personalidad (TLP)

Botulinum Toxin (Botox) *f.* Toxina Botulínica (Bótox)

Bound Morpheme *m.* Morfema Ligado

Brackets *m.* Corchetes

Bradykinesia *f.* Bradicinesia

Brainstem *m.* Tronco del Encéfalo; *m.* Tronco Encefálico

Breath Group *m.* Grupo del Respiro

Breathing Exercises *m.* Ejercicios Respiratorios; *m.* Ejercicios de Respiración

Breathy Voice *f.* Voz Entrecortada

Broad Transcription *f.* Transcripción Amplia

Broca's Aphasia *f.* Afasia de Broca

Broca's Area *m.* Área de Broca

Brodmann Areas *m.p.* Áreas de Brodmann

Bronchi *m.p.* Bronquios

Bronchioles *m.p.* Bronquiolos

Bruit *m.* Soplo

Buccal *a.* Bucal

Buccal Cavity *f.* Cavidad Bucal

Buccinator Muscle *m.* Músculo Buceador; *m.* Músculo Buccinador; *m.* Músculo Carrillo

Buccofacial Apraxia *f.* Apraxia Bucofacial

Bulbar *a.* Bulbar

Bulbar Palsy *f.* Parálisis Bulbar

Bulimia *f.* Bulimia

Bumpy Speech *f.* Habla Irregular; *f.* Habla Picada; *f.* Habla Entrecortada

C

Calcarine Sulcus *m*. Surco Calcarino; *f*. Fisura Calcarina

Calibrate *v*. Calibrar

Cancer *m*. Cáncer

Cancerous *a*. Canceroso -a

Cancerous Growth *m*. Crecimiento Canceroso

Candidacy *f*. Candidatura

Cannula *f*. Cánula

Cardiac *a*. Cardíaco-a

Cardiofaciocutaneous Syndrome (CFC) *m*. Síndrome Cardiofaciocutáneo (CFC)

Cardiopulmonary Resuscitation (CPR) *f*. Reanimación Cardiopulmonar (RCP)

Carotid Endarterectomy (CEA) *f*. Endarterectomía Carotídea (EAC)

Carryover *m*. Traspaso

Cartilage *m*. Cartílago

Case History *f*. Historia Clínica; *f*. Historia Médica

Caseload *f*. Carga de Trabajo; *f*. Carga de Casos; *f*. Carga de Pacientes

Case Marker *m*. Marcador de Caso

Case Study *m*. Estudio de Caso; *m*. Análisis de Caso

Catheter *m*. Catéter

Caudate Nucleus *m*. Núcleo Caudado

Cavity *f*. Cavidad

Centers for Disease Control and Prevention (CDC) *m.p* Centros Para el Control y la Prevención de Enfermedades (CDC)

Central Auditory Processing Disorder (CAPD) *m*. Trastorno del Procesamiento Auditivo Central (TPAC)

Central Nervous System (CNS) *m*. Sistema Nervioso Central (SNC)

Central Sulcus *m*. Surco Central; *f*. Cisura de Rolando

Central Vowel *f*. Vocal Central

Cerebellar *a*. Cerebelar

Cerebellum *m.* Cerebelo

Cerebrovascular Accident (CVA) *m.* Accidente Cerebrovascular (ACV); *m.* Ictus; *f.* Enfermedad Cerebrovascular (ECV); *m.* Infarto Cerebral

Cerebral Palsy *f.* Parálisis Cerebral

Cerebrospinal Fluid (CSF) *m.* Líquido Cerebroespinal (LCE); *m.* Líquido Cefalorraquídeo (LCR)

Cerebrum *m.* Cerebro

Certificate of Clinical Competence (CCC) *m.* Certificado de Competencia Clínica (CCC)

Certified *a.* Acreditado-a; *a.* Certificado-a

Certified Occupational Therapy Assistant (COTA) *m.* Asistente Certificado de Terapia Ocupacional (COTA)

Cerumen *m.* Cerumen

Cervical *a.* Cervical

Cervical Auscultation *f.* Auscultación Cervical

Cervical Collar *m.* Collarín Cervical

CHARGE Syndrome *m.* Síndrome CHARGE

Charitable Organization *f.* Organización Benéfica; *f.* Organización Caritativa

Charity *f.* Caridad

Chemotherapy *f.* Quimioterapia

Chiari Malformation *f.* Malformación de Chiari

Child Abuse *m.* Abuso Infantil

Child Protective Services (CPS) *m.p* Servicios de Protección de Niños (CPS)

Childhood Apraxia of Speech (CAS) *f.* Apraxia del Habla Infantil (CAS)

Chin Tuck *f.* Barbilla Hacia Abajo

Choanal Atresia *f.* Atresia Coanal

Chondral *a.* Condral

Chorea *f.* Corea

Choreoathetosis *f.* Coreoatetosis

Chromosomal Disorder *m.* Trastorno Cromosómico

Chromosome *m.* Cromosoma

Chronic *a.* Crónico -a

[31]

Chronic Obstructive Pulmonary Disease (COPD) *f.* Enfermedad Pulmonar Obstructiva Crónica (EPOC)

Chronic Traumatic Encephalopathy (CTE) *f.* Encefalopatía Traumática Crónica (ETC)

Chronological Age *f.* Edad Cronológica

Cilia *m.p.* Cilios; *f.p.* Cilias

Cingulate Gyrus *m.* Giro Cingulado

Circle of Willis *m.* Círculo Arterial Cerebral; *m.* Polígono de Willis

Circumlocution *m.* Circunloquio

Circumvallate Papillae *f.p* Papilas Circunvaladas; *f.p* Papilas Linguales

Claustrum *m.* Claustrum

Clavicle *f.* Clavícula

Cleft *f.* Hendidura

Cleft Lip *m.* Labio Leporino; *m.* Labio Hendido

Cleft Palate *m.* Paladar Hendido

Click Consonant *m.* Chasquido Consonántico

Clinical Fellow *m/f*. Becario-a Clínico-a

Clinical Fellowship *f*. Práctica Clínica; *m*. Posgrado Clínico; *m*. Internado Profesional

Close Vowel *f*. Vocal Cerrada; *f*. Vocal Alta

Closed Head Injury (CHI) *f*. Lesión Craneal Cerrada

Close-Mid Vowel *f*. Vocal Semicerrada

Closure *m*. Cierre

Clot *m*. Coágulo

Cluttering *m*. Lenguaje Apresurado; *m*. Lenguaje Precipitado; *m*. Balbuceo

Coaching *m*. Entrenamiento

Coalescence *f*. Coalescencia; *f*. Unión

Coarticulation *f*. Coarticulación

Coccyx *m*. Coxis; *m*. Cóccix

Cochlea *f*. Cóclea; *m*. Caracol

Cochlear Duct *f*. Rampa Coclear

Cochlear Implant *m*. Implante Coclear

Cochlear Nerve *m.* Nervio Coclear

Cochlear Nucleus *m.* Núcleo Coclear

Coda *f.* Coda

Code Switching *f.* Alternancia de Códigos; *m.* Cambio de Códigos

Codification *f.* Codificación

Cognate *m.* Cognado

Cognition *f.* Cognición

Cognitive Development *m.* Desarrollo Cognitivo

Cohesion *f.* Cohesión

Cohort Study *m.* Estudio de Cohorte

Coma *m.* Coma

Comatose *a.* Comatoso-a

Commissurotomy *f.* Comisurotomía

Common Carotid Artery *f.* Arteria Carótida Común

Common Cold *m.* Resfriado Común; *m.* Resfrío; *m.* Catarro; *m.* Constipado

Communicating Artery *f.* Arteria Comunicante

Communication Disorders *m.p* Trastornos de la Comunicación

Communication Sciences *f.p* Ciencias de la Comunicación

Communicative Competence *f.* Competencia Comunicativa

Communicative Intent *m.* Intento Comunicativo; *f.* Intención Comunicativa

Community *f.* Comunidad

Comorbid *a.* Comórbido-a

Comorbidity *f.* Comorbilidad

Compensatory Strategies *f.p* Estrategias Compensatorias

Compensatory Swallow *f.* Deglución Compensatoria

Completely in Canal Hearing Aid (CIC) *m.* Audífono Completamente en el Canal (CIC)

Comprehension *f.* Comprensión

Computed Tomography (CT) Scan *f.* Tomografía Computarizada (TC); *f.* Tomografía Axial Computarizada (TAC)

Conceptual Apraxia *f.* Apraxia Conceptual

Concrete Operational Stage *f.* Etapa Operacional Concreta

Concussion *f.* Concusión

Conditioning *m.* Condicionamiento

Conduction Aphasia *f.* Afasia de Conducción

Conductive Hearing Loss *f.* Pérdida Auditiva Conductiva

Confidence Interval *m.* Intervalo de Confianza

Confidentiality *f.* Confidencialidad

Confrontation Naming *m.* Nombramiento Solicitado

Congenital *a.* Congénito -a

Conjugation *f.* Conjugación

Consonant *f.* Consonante

Consonant Clusters *m.p* Grupos Consonánticos

Constipation *m.* Estreñimiento

Constructional Apraxia *f.* Apraxia Constructiva

Context *m.* Contexto

Contextualization *f.* Contextualización

Continuant *f.* Continuante

Continuing Care *m.* Cuidado Continuo

Continuing Education Unit (CEU) *f.* Unidad de Educación Continua (CEU)

Continuity *f.* Continuidad

Continous Positive Airway Pressure (CPAP) *f.* Presión Positiva Continua en la Vía Respiratoria (CPAP)

Continuum of Naturalness *m.* Continuo de Naturalidad

Contract *m.* Contrato

Contraction *f.* Contracción

Contrast *v.* Contrastar

Conversational Turn Taking *v.* Tomar Turnos en Conversación

Coo *v.* Arrullar

Cooing *m.* Arrullo

Cooperative Play *m.* Juego Cooperativo

Coordination *f.* Coordinación

Coprolalia *f.* Coprolalia

Cordectomy *f.* Cordectomía

Core Vocabulary *m.* Vocabulario Núcleo

Coronal *a.* Coronal

Corona Radiata *f.* Corona Radiata

Corpus Callosum *m.* Cuerpo Calloso

Correlation *f.* Correlación

Correlation Coefficient *m.* Coeficiente de Correlación

Cortex *f.* Corteza

Cortical *a.* Cortical

Cortical Arousal *m.* Arousal Cortical

Cortical Blindness *f.* Ceguera Cortical

Cortical Deafness *f.* Sordera Cortical

Corticobulbar Tract *m.* Tracto Corticobulbar

Corticospinal Tract *m.* Tracto Corticoespinal

Cough *f.* Tos

Counseling *m.* Asesoramiento

Counselor *m/f.* Consejero-a; *m/f.* Asesor-a

Cracker *f.* Galleta

Cranial *a.* Craneal

Cranial Nerve *m.* Par Craneal; *m.* Nervio Craneal

Craniectomy *f.* Craniectomía

Craniofacial Anomalies *f.p* Anomalías Craneofaciales

Craniotomy *f.* Craniotomía

Creole *m.* Creole; *f.* Lengua Criolla

Crest *f.* Cresta

Cricoarytenoid *a.* Cricoaritenoide

Cricoid Cartilage *m.* Cartílago Cricoides

Cricopharyngeal *a.* Cricofaríngeo -a

Cricothyroid *a.* Cricotiroideo

Criterion-Referenced Tests *f.p.* Pruebas Referidas a Criterios

Critical Period *m.* Periodo Crítico

Cue *f.* Señal

Cued Speech *f.* La Palabra Complementada (LPC)

Cueing *f.* Señalización

Cultural Background *m.* Contexto Cultural

Cultural Competence *f.* Competencia Cultural; *f.* Consciencia Cultural

Cyst *m.* Quiste

Cystic Fibrosis *f.* Fibrosis Quística

D

Data *m.* Datos

Deaf *a.* Sordo-a

Deafness *f.* Sordera

Decibel (dB) *m.* Decibelio (dB)

Decoding *f.* Descodificación

Decubitus *m.* Decúbito

Decussation *f.* Decusación

Deep Brain Stimulation (DBS) *f.* Estimulación Cerebral Profunda (DBS)

Degenerative *a.* Degenerativo-a

Deglutition *f.* Deglución

Degree *m.* Grado

Dehydrate *v.* Deshidratar

Dehydration *f.* Deshidratación

Deixis *f.* Deixis

Delay *m.* Retraso

Delayed *a.* Retardado -a; *a.* Retrasado -a

Deletion *f.* Supresión; *f.* Elisión

Dementia *f.* Demencia

Demyelinating *a.* Desmielinizante

Dendrite *f.* Dendrita

Dental *a.* Dental

Dental Arch *m.* Arco Dental

Dental Occlusion *f.* Oclusión Dental

Dentition *f.* Dentición

Deoxyribonucleic Acid (DNA) *m.* Ácido Desoxirribonucleico (ADN)

Department of Health and Human Services (DHHS) *m.* Departamento de Salud y Servicios Humanos (DHHS)

Depression *f.* Depresión

Dermatome *m.* Dermatoma

Descriptive Grammar *m.* Descriptivismo

Descriptivist *m/f.* Descriptivista

[42]

Deterioration *m.* Deterioro

Development *m.* Desarrollo

Developmental Age *f.* Edad de Desarrollo

Developmental Delay *m.* Retraso de Desarrollo

Developmental Language Disorder (DLD) *m.* Trastorno del Desarrollo del Lenguaje (TDL); *m.* Trastorno del Lenguaje (TDL)

Developmental Verbal Dyspraxia (DVD) *f.* Dispraxia Verbal del Desarrollo (DVD)

Device *m.* Dispositivo

Devoicing *m.* Ensordecimiento

Diabetes *f.* Diabetes

Diabetic *a.* Diabético -a

Diacritic Mark *m.* Símbolo Diacrítico

Diadochokinesis *f.* Diadococinesis

Diadochokinetic Rate *f.* Tasa Diadococinética'

Diaeresis *f.* Diéresis

Diagnose *v.* Diagnosticar

[43]

Diagnosis *m.* Diagnóstico

Dialect *m.* Dialecto

Dialysis *f.* Diálisis

Diaphragm *m.* Diafragma

Diaschisis *f.* Diasquisis

Didactic *a.* Didáctico-a

Diet *f.* Dieta; *f.* Alimentación; *m.* Régimen Alimentario

Dietary *a.* Dietético-a; *a.* Alimenticio-a

Dietary Intake *f.* Ingesta Dietética; *f.* Ingestión Alimenticia; *f.* Ingesta Alimentaria

Dietary Supplement *m.* Suplemento Dietético

Dietician *m/f.* Dietista

Diffuse Esophageal Spasm *m.* Espasmo Esofágico Difuso

Diffusion MRI *f.* IRM de Difusión

Digastric Muscle *m.* Músculo Digástrico

Digestion *f.* Digestión

Digestive System *m.* Sistema Digestivo

Digitized Speech *f.* Habla Digitalizada

Diglossia *f.* Diglosia

Digraph *m.* Dígrafo

Dilation *f.* Dilatación

Diminutive *m.* Diminutivo

Diphone *m.* Difono

Diphthong *m.* Diptongo

Diphthongization *f.* Diptongación

Disability *f.* Discapacidad

Discrimination *f.* Discriminación

Dislocation *f.* Dislocación

Displacement *m.* Desplazamiento

Dissimilation *f.* Disimilación

Distal *a.* Distal

Distinction *f.* Distinción

Diversity *f.* Diversidad

Diverticulum *m.* Divertículo

Dominant *a*. Dominante

Dopamine *f*. Dopamina

Dorsal *a*. Dorsal

Dorsal Root Ganglia *m.p*. Ganglios de las Raíces Dorsales; *m.p*. Ganglios Espinales

Dorsum *m*. Dorso

Down Syndrome *m*. Síndrome de Down

Dressing Apraxia *f*. Apraxia del Vestir

Drill *m*. Ejercicio

Drugs *m.p*. Medicamentos; *m.p*. Fármacos

Dura Mater *f*. Duramadre

Dynamic Aphasia *f*. Afasia Dinámica

Dynamic Assessment *f*. Evaluación Dinámica (ED)

Dysarthria *f*. Disartria

Dysexecutive Syndrome (DES) *m*. Síndrome Disejecutivo (SD)

Dysfluency *f*. Disfluencia; *f*. Disfluidez

Dysfunction *f.* Disfunción

Dysfunctional *a.* Disfuncional

Dysgraphia *f.* Disgrafía

Dyskinesia *f.* Discinesia

Dyslalia *f.* Dislalia

Dyslexia *f.* Dislexia

Dysorthography *f.* Disortografía

Dysostosis *f.* Disostosis

Dysphagia *f.* Disfagia

Dysphonia *f.* Disfonía

Dysplasia *f.* Displasia

Dyspnea *f.* Disnea

Dyspraxia *f.* Dispraxia

Dysprosody *f.* Disprosodia

Dystonia *f.* Distonía

Dystrophy *f.* Distrofia

E

Ear Canal *m*. Conducto Auditivo Externo (CAE); *m*. Meato Auditivo Externo

Ear Canal Volume (ECV) *m*. Volumen del Conducto Auditivo Externo (ECV)

Ear, Nose and Throat Practice (ENT) *f*. Clínica de Otorrinolaringología

Eardrum *m*. Tímpano; *f*. Membrana Timpánica; *f*. Caja Timpánica

Early Intervention *f*. Intervención Temprana; Intervención Rápida

Easy Onset *m*. Inicio Suave

Echolalia *f*. Ecolalia

Ectoderm *m*. Ectodermo

Edema *m*. Edema

Edentulous *a*. Edéntulo-a

Educational Environment *m*. Entorno Educativo; *m*. Ambiente Educativo

Efferent *a*. Eferente

Efficacy *f*. Eficacia

Electrical Potential *m*. Potencial Eléctrico

Electrocochleography **(ECoG)** *f*. Electrococleografía (ECoG)

Electrode *m*. Electrodo

Electroencephalography **(EEG)** *f*. Electroencefalografía (EEG)

Electroglottography (EGG) *m*. Laringógrafo (EGG)

Elementary School *f*. Escuela Primaria

Elide *v*. Elidir

Elision *f*. Elisión

Embolic Stroke *m*. Ictus Embólico

Embolism *f*. Embolia

Embolus *m*. Émbolo

Embryo *m*. Embrión

Embryonic *a*. Embrionario-a

[49]

Emotional Lability *f.* Labilidad Emocional

Empirical *a.* Empírico-a

Encephalitis *f.* Encefalitis

Encephalopathy *f.* Encefalopatía

Endodermo *m.* Endoderm

Endogenous *a.* Endógeno-a

Endolymph *f.* Endolinfa

Endolymphatic Hydrops *m.* Hidrops Endolinfático

Endoscope *m.* Endoscopio

Endoscopic Ultrasound *m.* Ultrasonido Endoscópico; *f.* Ecografía Endoscópica

English as a Foreign Language (EFL) *m.* Inglés Como Lengua Extranjera (EFL)

English as a Second Language (ESL) *m.* Inglés Como Segunda Lengua (ESL)

Enhanced Milieu Teaching (EMT) *f.* Enseñanza Ambiental Mejorada (EMT)

Enteral Nutrition *f.* Nutrición Enteral

Enzyme *f.* Enzima

Eosinophilic Esophagitis *f.* Esofagitis Eosinofílica

Epenthesis *f.* Epéntesis

Epidural *a.* Epidural

Epiglottic Petiole *m.* Tallo Epiglótico; *m.* Pecíolo Epiglótico

Epiglottis *f.* Epiglotis

Epilepsy *f.* Epilepsia

Episodic Memory *f.* Memoria Episódica

Epyndemal Cells *m.p.* Epéndimocitos; *f.p.* Células Ependimarias

Esophageal Atresia *f.* Atresia Esofágica

Esophageal Dysphagia *f.* Disfagia Esofágica

Esophageal Lumen *m.* Lumen Esofágico

Esophageal Manometry *f.* Manometría Esofágica

Esophageal Phase *f.* Fase Esofágica

Esophageal Ring *m.* Anillo Esofágico

Esophageal Stricture *m.* Estenosis Esofágico

Esophagectomy *f.* Esofagectomía

Esophagitis *f.* Esofagitis

Esophagus *m.* Esófago

Essential Tremor (ET) *m.* Temblor Esencial (TE)

Ethics *f.* Ética

Ethnographic *a.* Etnográfico-a

Ethnolinguistic *a.* Etnolingüístico-a

Etiology *f.* Etiología

Etymology *f.* Etimología

Eupnea *f.* Eupnea

Eustachian Tube *f.* Trompa de Eustaquio; *f.* Tuba; *m.* Tubo Faringotimpánico; *f.* Trompa Auditiva

Evaluation *f.* Evaluación

Evidence-Based Practice (EBP) *f.* Práctica Basada en la Evidencia (PBE)

Exacerbation *f.* Exacerbación

Executive Function *f*. Función Ejecutiva

Exogenous *a*. Exógeno-a

Expansion *f*. Expansión

Expectorate *v*. Expectorar

Expiration of Air *f*. Espiración de Aire

Explicit Memory *f*. Memoria Explícita

Expressive Aphasia *f*. Afasia Expresiva

Expressive Language *m*. Lenguaje Expresivo

Extend *v*. Extender

Extension *f*. Extensión

External *a*. Externo -a

External Auditory Meatus (EAM) *m*. Meato Auditivo Externo; *m*. Conducto Auditivo Externo (CAE)

Extrapyramidal *a*. Extrapiramidal

Eye Contact *m*. Contacto Visual

Eye Gaze *f*. Mirada

F

Facial Nerve *m.* Nervio Facial

Facilitate *v.* Facilitar

False Vocal Cords *f.p* Cuerdas Vocales Falsas

Family Therapy *f.* Terapia Familiar

Fasciculation *f.* Fasciculación

Fasciculus *m.* Fascículo

Fatigue *f.* Fatiga

Fauces *m.* Istmo de las Fauces

Faucial Arches *m.p* Arcos Fauciales

Feedback *m.* Feedback; *f.* Retroalimentación

Feeding *f.* Alimentación

Feeding Team *m.* Equipo de la Alimentación

Feeding Therapist *m/f.* Terapeuta de la Alimentación

Fetal *a.* Fetal

Fetal Alcohol Syndrome (FAS) *m.* Síndrome Alcohólico Fetal (SAF)

Fetus *m.* Feto

Fiberoptic Endoscopic Evaluation of Swallowing (FEES) *f.* Evaluación Endoscópica de la Deglución por Fibra Óptica (FEES)

Fiberscope *m.* Fibroscopio

Figurative Language *m.* Lenguaje Figurativo

Filler *f.* Muletilla

Final Consonant Deletion *f.* Supresión de Consonantes Finales

Fine Motor Skills *f.* Motricidad Fina

Finger Agnosia *f.* Agnosia Digital

Fingerspelling *m.* Alfabeto Manual

Fissure *f.* Cisura ; *f.* Fisura ; *m.* Surco

Fissure of Rolando *f.* Cisura de Rolando ; *m.* Surco Central

Fistula *f.* Fístula

Flaccid Dysarthria *f.* Disartria Flácida

Flaccidity *f.* Flacidez

Flap *f.* Vibrante Simple

Flex *v.* Flexionar

Flexible Endoscopic Evaluation of Swallowing with Sensory Testing (FEESST) *f.* La Evaluación Endoscópica Flexible de la Deglución con Pruebas Sensoriales (FEESST)

Flexion *f.* Flexión

Floor of the Mouth *f.* Base de la Boca; *m.* Piso de la Boca

Fluency *f.* Fluidez

Fluency Shaping *f.* Modelación de la Fluidez

Fluency of Speech *f.* Fluidez del Habla

Fluent *a.* Fluido-a

Fluent Aphasia *f.* Afasia Fluente

Fluid *m.* Líquido

Fluoroscopy *f.* Fluoroscopia

Food and Drug Administration (FDA) *f.* Administración de Alimentos y Medicamentos (FDA)

Foramen *m.* Foramen; *m.* Agujero

Foramen Magnum *m.* Agujero Magno; *m.* Foramen Magno; *m.* Agujero Occipital

Forebrain *m.* Prosencéfalo

Foreign Bodies *m.* Cuerpos Extranjeros; *m.* Materiales Extranjeros

Formal Operational Stage *f.* Etapa Operacional Formal

Formant *m.* Formante

Formative Assessment *f.* Evaluación Formativa

Formulaic Language *m.* Lenguaje Formuláico

Fortition *f.* Fortición

Fragile X Syndrome (FXS) *m.* Síndrome del Cromosoma X Frágil (SFX)

Free Morpheme *m.* Morfema Libre

Freidreich's Ataxia *f.* Ataxia de Freidreich

Frenum *m.* Frenillo

Frequency *f.* Frecuencia

Frequency of Occurrence *f.* Frecuencia de Aparición

Fricative *f.* Fricativa; *a.* Fricativo-a

Front Vowel *f.* Vocal Anterior

Frontal Eye Field *m.* Campo Ocular Frontal

Frontal Lobe *m.* Lóbulo Frontal

Frontotemporal Dementia (FTD) *f.* Demencia Frontotemporal (DFT)

Frontotemporal Lobar Degeneration (FTLD) *f.* Degeneración Lobular Frontotemporal (DLFT)

Fronted *a.* Anteriorizado-a; *a.* Adelantado-a

Frontedness *f.* Anterioridad

Fronting *f.* Anteriorización

Functional *a.* Funcional

Functional Language *m.* Lenguaje Funcional

Functional Magnetic Resonance Imaging (fMRI) *f.* Imagen por Resonancia Magnética Funcional (IRMf)

Fundamental Frequency *f.* Frecuencia Fundamental

Fusiform Gyrus *m.* Giro Fusiforme

G

Gag Reflex *m.* Reflejo Nauseoso

Gait *f.* Andadura

Gait Apraxia *f.* Apraxia de la Marcha

Gamma-Aminobutyric Acid (GABA) *m.* Ácido Gamma-Aminobutírico (GABA)

Gastric *a.* Gástrico-a

Gastric Reflux *m.* Reflujo Gástrico

Gastroesophageal *a.* Gastroesofágico-a

Gastroesophageal Reflux Disease (GERD) *f.* Enfermedad del Reflujo Gastroesofágico (ERGE)

Gastrostomy *f.* Gastrostomía

Gavage *f.* Sonda Gástrica; *f.* Sonda Nasogástrica

Gemination *f.* Geminación

Gender-Neutral *a.* Neutral en Cuanto al Género

Gendered *a.* De Género

Gene *m.* Gen

Generalize *v.* Generalizar

Generalized Anxiety Disorder (GAD) *m.* Trastorno de Ansiedad Generalizada (TAG)

Generative Grammar *f.* Gramática Generativa

Generic *a.* Genérico-a

Genetic *a.* Genético-a

Geriatric *a.* Geriátrico-a

Gestalt *m.* Gestalt

Gestation *f.* Gestación

Gestational Age *f.* Edad Gestacional

Gesture *m.* Gesto

Gingiva *f.p.* Encías

Gland *f.* Glándula

Glasgow Coma Scale (GCS) *f.* Escala de Coma de Glasgow

Glial Cells *f.p.* Células Gliales

Glided *a.* Deslizado-a

Glide *f.* Deslizada; *f.* Semivocal

Gliding *m*. Deslizamiento

Glioma *m*. Glioma

Global Aphasia *f*. Afasia Global

Globus *m*. Globo

Globus Pallidus *m*. Globo Pálido

Globus Sensation *f*. Sensación de Globo

Glossectomy *f*. Glosectomía

Glossolalia *f*. Glosolalia

Glossopharyngeal Breathing *f*. Respiración Glosofaríngea

Glossopharyngeal Nerve *m*. Nervio Glosofaríngeo

Glottal *a*. Glotal

Glottal Fry *m*. Registro Glotal

Glottis *f*. Glotis

Goal *f*. Meta; *m*. Objetivo

Graft *m*. Injerto

Grammar *f*. Gramática

Grapheme *f*. Grafema

Gray Matter *f.* Sustancia Gris

Gross Motor Skills *f.* Motricidad Gruesa

Guillain–Barré Syndrome (GBS) *m.* Síndrome de Guillain-Barré

Gums *f.p.* Encías

Gunshot Wound (GSW) *f.* Herida por Arma de Fuego

Gyrus *m.* Giro

H

Habilitation *f.* Habilitación

Hallucination *f.* Alucinación

Hair Cells *f.p.* Células Ciliadas

Handicap *m.* Hándicap; *f.* Desventaja

Hard Glottal Attack *m.* Ataque Vocal Duro; *m.* Golpe Glótico

Hard Palate *m.* Paladar Duro

Head and Neck Cancer *m.* Cáncer de Cabeza y Cuello

Health Literacy *f.* Alfabetización en Salud

Hearing *f.* Audición

Hearing Aid *m.* Audífono

Hearing Impairment *f.* Discapacidad Auditiva

Hearing Loss *f.* Pérdida Auditiva

Heart Attack *m.* Infarto; *m.* Ataque Cardiaco; *m.* Ataque al Corazón; *m.* Infarto Agudo de Miocardio (IAM)

Heartburn *f.* Acidez

Hebbian Theory *f.* Teoría Hebbiana

Helicotrema *m.* Helicotrema

Helix *f.* Hélice

Hemianopsia *f.* Hemianopsia

Hemiballism *m.* Hemibalismo

Hemiparesis *f.* Hemiparesia

Hemiplegia *f.* Hemiplejia

Hemispatial Neglect *m.* Trastorno de Omisión; *m.* Hemiomisión; *m.* Síndrome Neurológico de la Desatención

Hemisphere (Left or Right) *m.* Hemisferio (Izquierdo o Derecho)

Hemorrhage *f.* Hemorragia

Hemorrhagic Stroke *m.* Ictus Hemorrágico

Hereditary *a.* Hereditario-a

Heritage Speaker *m.* Hablante de Herencia

Hernia *f.* Hernia

Hertz (Hz) *m.* Hercio (Hz)

Heschl's Gyrus *m.* Giro de Heschl; *m.* Giro Temporal Transverso

Heterogeneous *a.* Heterogéneo-a

Hiatus *m.* Hiato

Hiccup *m.* Hipo

High Blood Pressure *f.* Presión Alta; *f.* Hipertensión

High School *f.* Preparatoria; *f.* Escuela Secundaria

High Vowel *f.* Vocal Cerrada; *f.* Vocal Alta

Hindbrain *m.* Rombencéfalo

HIPAA Policy *f.* Política de Privacidad de HIPAA

Hippocampus *m.* Hipocampo

Hoarseness *f.* Ronquera

Holistic *a.* Holístico-a

Holoprosencephaly (HPE) *f.* Holoprosencefalia (HPE)

Home Health Care *f.* Atención Médica Domiciliaria; *m.* Cuidados Domiciliarios; *m.* Cuidado en Casa

Homeostasis *f.* Homeostasis

Homogenous *a.* Homogéneo-a

Homunculus *m.* Homúnculo

Honey *f.* Miel

Hospice *m.* Hospicio

Hospitalization *f.* Hospitalización

House Call *f.* Visita en Domicilio

Human Immunodeficiency Virus (HIV) *m.* Virus de la Inmunodeficiencia Humana (VIH)

Huntington's Disease (HD) *f.* Enfermedad de Huntington (EH)

Hydrocephalus *f.* Hidrocefalia

Hyoid Bone *m.* Hueso Hioides

Hypercorrection *f.* Hipercorrección

Hyperflexion *f.* Hiperflexión

Hyperkinesia *f.* Hipercinesia

Hyperkinetic *a.* Hipercinético-a

Hyperkinetic Dysarthria *f.* Disartria Hipercinética

Hypernasal *a.* Hipernasal

Hyperperfusion *f.* Hiperperfusión

Hyperreflexion *f.* Hiperreflexión

Hypertension (HTN) *f.* Hipertensión (HTN); *f.* Presión Alta

Hyperthyroidism *m.* Hipertiroidismo

Hypertonia *f.* Hipertonía

Hypertonic *a.* Hipertónico-a

Hypoglossal Nerve *m.* Nervio Hipogloso

Hypokinesia *f.* Hipocinesia

Hypokinetic Dysarthria *f.* Disartria Hipocinética

Hyponasal *a.* Hiponasal

Hypoperfusion *f.* Hipoperfusión

Hypopharyngeal Diverticula *m.p* Divertículos de la Hipofaringe

Hypopharynx *f.* Hipofaringe

Hypothalamus *m.* Hipotálamo

Hypothesis *f.* Hipótesis

Hypothyroidism *m.* Hipotiroidismo

Hypotonic *a.* Hipotónico-a

Hypoxia *f.* Hipoxia

I

Ideomotor Apraxia *f.* Apraxia Ideomotora

Idiolect *m.* Idiolecto

Idiom *m.* Idiotismo

Idiomatic *a.* Idiomático-a

Idiosyncratic *a.* Idiosincrático-a

Ilium *m.* Ilion

Illiteracy *m.* Analfabetismo

Illiterate *a.* Analfabeto-a

Illocutionary *a.* Ilocutivo-a

Imaging *f.p.* Imágenes

Imitation *f.* Imitación

Immersion Education *f.* Educación por Inmersión

Immittance *f.* Inmitancia

Immunity *f.* Inmunidad

Immunization *f.* Inmunización

Impaction (of Cerumen) *m.* Exceso (de Cerumen)

Impairment *m.* Deterioro; *f.* Discapacidad

Impedance *f.* Impedancia

Impedianciometry *f.* Impedanciometría

Implicit Memory *f.* Memoria Implícita

Improvement *f.* Mejora; *f.* Mejoría; *m.* Avance

In the Ear Hearing Aid (ITE) *m.* Audífono Intrauricular (ITE)

Incidence *f.* Incidencia

Incidental Teaching *f.* Enseñanza Incidental

Incisors *m.p* Incisivos

Inclusion *f.* Inclusión; *f.* Integración

Incompetence *f.* Incompetencia

Incus *m.* Yunque

Individualized Education Program (IEP) *m.* Programa de Educación Individualizado

Individuals with Disabilities Education Act (IDEA) *f.* Ley Para la Educación de Individuos con Discapacidades (IDEA)

Induction *f.* Inducción

Infant *m.* Infante

Infantile *a.* Infantil

Infarct *m.* Infarto

Infection *f.* Infección

Inferior Colliculus *m.* Colículo Inferior

Inflammation *f.* Inflamación

Inflection *f.* Flexión

Infrahyoid Muscles *m.p* Músculos Infrahioideos

Inhale *v.* Inhalar

Inhaler *m.* Inhalador

Inherit *v.* Heredar

Inherited *a.* Heredado-a

Initial Consonant Deletion *f.* Supresión de Consonantes Iniciales

[71]

Injection *f.* Inyección

Injury *m.* Traumatismo; *f.* Lesión; *f.* Herida

Innate *a.* Innato-a

Inner Ear *m.* Oído Interno

Innervation *f.* Inervación

Inpatient *a.* Hospitalario-a; *a.* Intrahospitalario-a

Inspire Air *v.* Inspirar Aire

Insula *f.* Ínsula

Intellectual Disability (ID) *f.* Discapacidad Intelectual

Intelligibility *f.* Inteligibilidad

Intensity *f.* Intensidad

Intensive Care Unit (ICU) *f.* Unidad de Cuidados Intensivos (UCI)

Intensive Therapy *f.* Terapia Intensiva

Intention Tremor *m.* Temblor Intencional

Interactionist *a.* Interaccionista

Interchangeability *f.* Intercambiabilidad

Interdental *a.* Interdental

Interference *f.* Interferencia

Interfix *m.* Interfijo

Interjection *f.* Interjección

Interlanguage *f.* Interlengua

Interlocutor *m/f.* Interlocutor-a

Intermediate *a.* Intermedio-a

Intermediate Care *f.* Atención Intermedia; *m.* Cuidado Intermedio

Intermittent *a.* Recurrente; *a.* Intermitente

Internal *a.* Interno -a

Internal Capsule *f.* Cápsula Interna

International Phonetic Alphabet (IPA) *m.* Alfabeto Fonético Internacional (AFI)

Interpreter *m/f.* Intérprete

Intervention *f.* Intervención

Interview *f.* Entrevista

Intonation *f.* Entonación

Intracranial Pressure (ICP) *f.* Presión Intracraneal (PIC)

Invasive *a.* Invasivo-a

Inventory *m.* Inventario

Irreversible *a.* Irreversible

Ischemia *f.* Isquemia

Ischemic Stroke *m.* Ictus Isquémico

Ischium *m.* Isquion

Isolation *m.* Aislamiento

J

Jargon *f.* Jerga

Jaw *f.* Mandíbula

Jitter *m.* Jitter; *f.* Fluctuación

Joint *f.* Articulación

K

Keratosis *f.* Queratosis

Kindergarten *m.* Kindergarten; *m.* Jardín de Infantes; *f.* Guardería

Kinesiologist *m/f.* Quinesiólogo-a; *m/f.* Kinesiólogo-a

Kinesiology *f.* Quinesiología; *f.* Kinesiología

Knowledge *m.* Conocimiento

Kyphosis *f.* Cifosis

L

Labeling *f.* Marcación

Labia *m.p.* Labios

Labial *a.* Labial

Labialization *f.* Labialización

Labiodental *a.* Labiodental

Labiovelar *a.* Labiovelar

Labyrinthitis *f.* Laberintitis

Lactation *f.* Lactación

Lamina *f.* Lámina

Laminal *f.* Laminar; *f.* Laminal

Language *m.* Lenguaje; *m.* Idioma; *f.* Lengua

Language Barriers *f.p* Barreras Lingüísticas; *f.p* Barreras Idiomáticas

Language Delay *m.* Retraso del Lenguaje; *m.* Trastorno del Desarrollo del Lenguaje; *m.* Trastorno del Lenguaje

Language Disorder *m*. Trastorno del Lenguaje; *m*. Trastorno del Desarrollo del Lenguaje

Language Sample *f*. Muestra de Lenguaje

Laryngeal *a*. Laríngeo-a

Laryngeal Dystonia *f*. Distonía Laríngea; *f*. Disfonía Espasmódica (SD)

Laryngeal Mask Airway (LMA) *f*. Vía Aérea con Mascarilla Laríngea (VAML)

Laryngeal Stroboscopy *f*. Estroboscopia Laríngea

Laryngeal Tube *m*. Tubo Laríngeo

Laryngectomy *f*. Laringectomía

Laryngitis *f*. Laringitis

Laryngocele *m*. Laringocele

Laryngologist *m/f*. Laringólogo

Laryngomalacia *f*. Laringomalacia

Laryngopharyngeal Reflux *m*. Reflujo Laringofaríngeo

Laryngoplasty *f*. Laringoplastia

Laryngoscope *m*. Laringoscopio

Laryngoscopy *f.* Laringoscopía

Laryngospasm *m.* Laringoespasmo

Larynx *f.* Laringe

Laser *m.* Láser

Late Language Emergence (LLE) *f.* Aparición Tardía del Lenguaje (LLE)

Late Talker *m.* Hablante Tardío

Lateral *f.* Lateral; *a.* Lateral

Lateral Geniculate Nucleus *m.* Núcleo Geniculado Lateral; *m.* Cuerpo Geniculado Lateral

Lateral Sulcus *m.* Surco Lateral; *f.* Cisura de Silvio

Laterality *f.* Lateralidad

Lax Vowel *f.* Vocal Laxa

Learned Behavior *m.* Comportamiento Aprendido

Learning *m.* Aprendizaje

Learning Disability (LD) *f.* Discapacidad del Aprendizaje; *f.* Dificultad en el Aprendizaje

Learning Style *m.* Estilo de Aprendizaje

Least Restrictive Environment *m.* Ambiente Menos Restrictivo

Lemma *m.* Lema

Lemniscus *m.* Lemnisco

Lenition *f.* Lenición

Lesion *f.* Lesión

Leukoplakia *f.* Leucoplasia

Levelling *f.* Nivelación

Lewy Bodies *m.p.* Cuerpos de Lewy

Lewy Body Dementia (LBD) *f.* Demencia con Cuerpos de Lewy (DCL)

Lexical *a.* Léxico-a

Lexicon *m.* Léxico

Ligament *m.* Ligamento

Limbic System *m.* Sistema Límbico

Limb-Kinetic Apraxia *f.* Apraxia de Extremidad Cinética

Limitation *f.* Limitación

Limited English Proficiency (LEP) *m.* Dominio Limitado del Inglés (LEP)

Ling Six Sounds *m.p.* Seis Sonidos de Ling

Lingua Franca *f.* Lingua Franca

Lingual *a.* Lingual

Linguistic Aspects *m.p.* Aspectos Lingüísticos

Linguistic Competence *f.* Competencia Lingüística

Linguistic Performance *m.* Desempeño Lingüístico

Linguistics *f.* Lingüística

Linguolabial Consonant *f.* Consonante Linguolabial

Lip Reading *f.* Lectura Labial

Liquid *f.* Líquida; *a.* Líquido-a

Lisp *m.* Ceceo

Lissencephaly *f.* Lisencefalia

Listener *m.* Oyente

Literacy *f.* Alfabetización

Literate *a.* Alfabetizado-a

Loan Word *m.* Préstamo

Lobe *m.* Lóbulo

Localization *f.* Localización

Logopedics *f.* Logopedia

Logopenic PPA *f.* APP Logopénica

Logorrhea *f.* Logorrea; *f.* Verborrea

Longitudinal *a.* Longitudinal

Longitudinal Fissure *f.* Cisura Interhemisférica; *f.* Cisura Intercerebral ; *f.* Cisura Longitudinal

Longitudinal Study *m.* Estudio Longitudinal

Long Vowel *f.* Vocal Larga

Long-Term Care *m.* Cuidado Prolongado; *f.* Atención a Largo Plazo; *m.* Cuidado a Larga Duración

Long-Term Memory (LTM) *f.* Memoria a Largo Plazo (MLP)

Lordosis *f.* Lordosis

Low Vowel *f.* Vocal Baja; *f.* Vocal Abierta

Lower *a.* Inferior

Lower Esophageal Sphincter (LES) *m.* Esfínter Esofágico
Inferior (EEI)

Lower Motor Neuron (LMN) *f.* Neurona Motora Inferior
(NMI)

Lowered *a.* Descendido-a

Lumen *m.* Lumen

Lungs *m.* Pulmones

Lymph *f.* Linfa

M

Macrocephaly *f.* Macrocefalia

Macroglossia *f.* Macroglosia

Magnetic Resonance Imaging (MRI) *f.* Imagen por Resonancia Magnética (IRM); *f.* Tomografía por Resonancia Magnética (TRM)

Mainstreaming *f.* Incorporación

Maladaptive *a.* Inadaptado-a

Malformation *f.* Malformación

Malignant *a.* Maligno-a

Malleus *m.* Martillo

Malocclusion *f.* Maloclusión

Mandible *f.* Mandíbula

Mandibular *a.* Mandibular

Mandibulofacial *a.* Mandibulofacial

Mand-Model Approach *m.* Modelo Mand

Manner of Articulation *m.* Modo de Articulación

Manometer *m.* Manómetro

Manual Alphabet *m.* Alfabeto Manual

Mapping *m.* Mapeo

Marginal Babbling *m.* Balbuceo Marginal

Marked *a.* Marcado-a

Masking *f.* Ocultación

Masseter Muscle *m.* Músculo Masetero

Masticated *a.* Masticado -a

Mastication *f,* Masticación

Mastoid *a.* Mastoideo-a

Maxilla *m.* Maxilar

Mean Length of Utterance (MLU) *f.* Talla Media de la Expresión (MLU)

Mean Value *m.* Valor Medio

Medial *a.* Medial

Medial Consonant Deletion *f.* Supresión de Consonantes Mediales

Medial Geniculate Nucleus *m.* Núcleo Geniculado Medial; *m.* Cuerpo Geniculado Lateral

Mediastinum *m.* Mediastino

Medulla Oblongata *m.* Bulbo Raquídeo; *f.* Médula Oblonga

Melodic Intonation Therapy (MIT) *f.* Terapia de Entonación Melódica (TEM)

Membrane *f.* Membrana

Membranous *a.* Membranoso-a

Memory *f.* Memoria

Memory Loss *f.* Pérdida de Memoria

Ménière's Disease (MD) *f.* Enfermedad de Ménière ; *m.* Síndrome de Ménière

Meninge *f.* Meninge

Meningitis *f.* Meningitis

Mental Age *f.* Edad Mental

Mentor *m.* Mentor

Mesencephalon *m.* Mesencéfalo

Mesoderm *m.* Mesodermo

Mesothelial *a.* Mesotelial

Mesothelioma *m.* Mesotelioma

Metabolism *m.* Metabolismo

Metacognition *f.* Metacognición

Metalinguistic *a.* Metalingüístico-a

Metaphor *f.* Metáfora

Metastasis *f.* Metástasis

Metathesis *f.* Metátesis'

Metencephalon *m.* Metencéfalo

Microcephaly *f.* Microcefalia

Microglia *f.p.* Microglía

Micrognathia *f.* Micrognacia

Microscope *m.* Microscopio

Microscopic *a.* Microscópico-a

Microsomia *f.* Microsomía

Microtia *f.* Microtia

Midbrain *m.* Mesencéfalo

Mid Vowel *f.* Vocal Intermedia

Middle Cerebral Artery (MCA) *f.* Arteria Cerebral Media (ACM)

Middle Ear *m.* Oído Medio

Middle School *f.* Escuela Secundaria; *f.* Intermedia

Midsagittal *a.* Mediano-a; *a.* Mediosagital; *a.* Medial

Migraine *f.* Migraña; *f.* Jaqueca; *f.* Hemicránea

Mild *a.* Leve

Mild Cognitive Impairment (MCI) *m.* Deterioro Cognitivo Leve (DCL)

Milieu Therapy *f.* Terapia Milieu ; *f.* Terapia Ambiental

Minimal Pair *m.* Par Mínimo

Minimally Invasive *a.* Mínimamente Invasivo-a

Minority *f.* Minoría

Misaligned *a.* Desalineado-a

Misalignment *f.* Desalineación

Mitigate *v.* Mitigar

Misarticulation *m.p* Errores de Articulación

Mixed Dysarthria *f.* Disartria Mixta

Mixed Hearing Loss *f.* Pérdida Auditiva Mixta

Mixed Transcortical Aphasia (MTA/MTCA) *f.* Afasia Transcortical Mixta

Modality *f.* Modalidad

Modeling *f.* Modelación

Moderate *a.* Moderado-a

Modified Barium Swallow Study (MBSS) *f.* Deglución de Bario (MBSS)

Modiolus *m.* Modiolo

Molars *m.* Molares

Monolingual *a.* Monolingüe

Monologue *m.* Monólogo

Monosyllabic *a.* Monosilábico-a

Morbidity *f.* Morbilidad

Morpheme *m.* Morfema

Morphology *f.* Morfología

Motherese *m.* Maternés

Motor Skills *f.* Motricidad; *f.* Motilidad

Motor Apraxia *f.* Apraxia Motriz

Motor Cortex *f.* Corteza Motora

Motor Learning *m.* Aprendizaje Motor

Motor Neuron *f.* Motoneurona; *f.* Neurona Motora; *f.* Neurona Motriz

Motor Neurone Disease (MND) *f.* Enfermedad de la Neurona Motora

Motor Speech Disorder *m.* Trastorno Motor del Habla

Motor Vehicle Accident (MVA) *f.* Accidente de Vehículo de Motor (AVM)

Movement *m.* Movimiento

Mucosa *f.* Mucosa

Mucous Membrane *f.* Membrana Mucosa

Multilingual *a.* Multilingüe; *a.* Plurilingüe

Multimodality *f*. Multimodalidad

Multiple Sclerosis (MS) *f*. Esclerosis Múltiple

Muscle *m*. Músculo

Muscle Tension Dysphonia *f*. Disfonía de Tensión Muscular

Muscle Tone *m*. Tono Muscular

Muscular Dystrophy (MD) *f*. Distrofia Muscular

Mutation *f*. Mutación

Mute *a*. Mudo-a

Mutism *m*. Mutismo

Myasthenia Gravis (MG) *f*. Miastenia Grave (MG)

Myelencephalon *m*. Mielencéfalo

Myelin *f*. Mielina

Myelin Sheath *f*. Vaina de Mielina

Myocardial Infarction (MI) *m*. Infarto de Miocardio (IM); *m*. Infarto

Myoclonus *m*. Mioclono

Myofascial Release *f*. Liberación Miofascial

Myofunctional *a*. Miofuncional

Myoneural Junction *f*. Unión Mioneural; *f*. Unión Neuromuscular

Myotome *m*. Miotoma

Myotomy *f*. Miotomía

Myringotomy *f*. Miringotomía

N

Naming *m.* Nombramiento

Narrative *f.* Narración

Narrow Transcription *f.* Transcripción Detallada

Nasal *f.* Nasal; *a.* Nasal

Nasal Cavity *f.* Cavidad Nasal

Nasal Emission *f.* Emisión Nasal

Nasality *f.* Nasalidad

Nasalization *f.* Nasalización

Nasogastric (NG) *a.* Nasogástrico-a (NG)

Nasogastric Feeding *f.* Alimentación Nasogástrica

Nasometry *f.* Nasometría

Nasopharynx *f.* Nasofaringe

National Association for Bilingual Education (NABE) *f.*
Asociación Nacional para la Educación Bilingüe (NABE)

National Dysphagia Diet (NDD) *f.* Dieta Nacional de
Disfagia (DND)

Native *a.* Nativo-a

Nativist *a.* Nativista

Nativization *f.* Nativización

Naturalist *a.* Naturalista

Near-Back Vowel *f.* Vocal Semiposterior

Near-Close Vowel *f.* Vocal Casicerrada

Near-Front Vowel *f.* Vocal Semianterior

Near-Open Vowel *f.* Vocal Casiabierta

Necrosis *f.* Necrosis

Nectar *m.* Néctar

Negation *f.* Negación

Negative Reinforcement *m.* Refuerzo Negativo; *m.* Reforzamiento Negativo

Neglect *f.* Negligencia; *m.* Abandono

Neonatal *a.* Neonatal

Neonatal Intensive Care Unit (NICU) *f.* Unidad de Cuidados Intensivos Neonatales (UCIN)

Neoplasm *f.* Neoplasia

Nerve *m.* Nervio

Nervous System *m.* Sistema Nervioso

Neural Tube *m.* Tubo Neural

Neural Tube Defect (NTD) *m.* Defecto del Tubo Neural (DTN)

Neurodegenerative *a.* Neurodegenerativo-a

Neurodiversity *f.* Neurodiversidad

Neurogenesis *f.* Neurogénesis

Neurolinguistics *f.* Neurolingüística

Neurological Damage *m.* Daño Neurológico

Neurologist *m/f.* Neurólogo-a

Neuromuscular Junction *f.* Unión Neuromuscular; *f.* Unión Mioneural

Neuron *f.* Neurona

Neuroplasticity *f.* Neuroplasticidad

Neurotransmitter *m.* Neurotransmisor; *m.* Neuromediador

Neurotypical *a.* Neurotípico-a

Neurulation *f.* Neurulación

Neutral *a.* Neutral

Neutralization *f.* Neutralización

Neutralize *v.* Neutralizar

Node *m.* Ganglio; *m.* Nodo

Node of Ranvier *m.* Nodo de Ranvier

Nodule *m.* Nódulo

Noise-Induced Hearing Loss *f.* Pérdida Auditiva Inducida por Ruido

Nonfluent Aphasia *f.* Afasia No Fluente

Nonfluent PPA *f.* APP No Fluente; *f.* APP Agramática

Nonprofit Organization (NPO) *f.* Organización Sin Fines de Lucro (OSFL); *f.* Organización Sin Ánimo de Lucro (OSAL); *f.* Organización No Lucrativa (ONL)

Nonverbal *a.* No Verbal

Norm-Referenced Tests *f.p.* Pruebas Referidas a la Norma

Normal Pressure Hydrocephalus (NPH) *f.* Hidrocefalia Normotensiva (HNT); *f.* Hidrocefalia Crónica del Adulto (HCA)

Normative *a.* Normativo-a

Nothing by Mouth/Nil per os (NPO) *a.* Nada por Vía Oral/Nil per os (NPO)

Notochord *f.* Notocorda; *m.* Notocordio

Nucleus *m.* Núcleo; *m.* Cuerpo

Null Hypothesis *f.* Hipótesis Nula

Nursing Home *m.* Geriátrico

Nutrition *f.* Nutrición

Nystagmus *m.* Nistagmo

O

Object Permanence *f.* Permanencia de los Objetos

Observation *f.* Observación

Observational Assessment *f.* Evaluación Observacional

Obstruct *v.* Obstruir

Obstruction *f.* Obstrucción

Obstruent *f.* Obstruyente; *a.* Obstruyente

Obturator *m.* Obturador

Occlusion *f.* Oclusión

Occlusive *f.* Oclusiva; *a.* Oclusivo-a

Occlusive Stroke *m.* Ictus Isquémico

Occupational Therapist *m/f.* Terapeuta Ocupacional

Occupational Therapy *f.* Terapia Ocupacional

Oculomotor Nerve *m.* Nervio Oculomotor; *m.* Nervio Motor Ocular Común (MOC)

Oculopharyngeal Muscular Dystrophy *f.* Distrofia Muscular Oculofaríngea

Odynophagia *f.* Odinofagia

Olfaction *m.* Olfato; *f.* Olfacción

Olfactory Bulb *m.* Bulbo Olfativo; *m.* Bulbo Olfatorio

Olfactory Nerve *m.* Nervio Olfativo; *m.* Nervio Olfatorio

Oligodendrocyte *m.* Oligodendrocito

Olivopontocerebellar Atrophy- OPCA *f.* Atrofia Olivopontocerebelosa (OPCA)

Omission *f.* Omisión

Onomatopoeia *f.* Onomatopeya

Onset *m.* Ataque; *m.* Inicio; *f.* Cabeza

Open Bite *f.* Mordida Abierta

Open Head Injury (OHI) *f.* Lesión Craneal Abierta

Open Vowel *f.* Vocal Abierta; *f.* Vocal Baja

Opening *f.* Abertura

Open-Mid Vowel *f.* Vocal Semiabierta

Operating Room (OR) *m.* Quirófano

Opercular Part *f.* Parte Opercular

Optic Chiasm *m.* Quiasma Óptico

Optic Nerve *m.* Nervio Ocular; *m.* Nervio Óptico

Oral Cavity *f.* Cavidad Oral; *f.* Cavidad Bucal

Oral Motor *a.* Motora Oral

Oral Peripheral Examination *m.* Examen Periférico Oral

Oral Phase *a.* Fase Oral

Oral Preparatory Phase *f.* Fase Oral Preparatoria

Oral Resonance *f.* Resonancia Oral

Orbicularis Oris Muscle *m.* Músculo Orbicular de la Boca

Organ of Corti *m.* Órgano de Corti; *m.* Órgano Espiral

Organic Disorder *m.* Trastorno Orgánico

Orofacial *a.* Orofacial

Orofacial Myofunctional Disorder (OMD) *m.* Trastorno Miofuncional Orofacial (OMD)

Orogastric *a.* Orogástrico-a

Oronasal *a.* Oronasal

Oropharyngeal Dysphagia *f.* Disfagia Orofaríngea

Oropharynx *f.* Orofaringe

Orthography *f.* Ortografía

Oscillation *f.* Oscilación

Osseus *a.* Óseo-a

Osseous Spiral Lamina *f.* Lámina Espiral Ósea

Ossicle *m.* Huesecillo

Ossicular Chain *f.* Cadena Osicular

Osteophyte *m.* Osteofito

Otitis Media (Acute/ Chronic) *f.* Otitis Media (Aguda/ Crónica)

Otoacoustic Emission (OAE) *f.* Emisión Otoacústica (EOA)

Otolith *m.* Otolito

Otologist *m/f.* Otólogo

Otorhinolaryngologist *m/f.* Otorrinolaringólogo

Otoscope *m.* Otoscopio

Otoscopy *f.* Otoscopia

Ototoxic *a.* Ototóxico-a

Outcome *m.* Resultado

Outer Ear *m.* Oído Externo

Outpatient *a.* Ambulatorio-a; *a.* Extrahospitalario-a

Oval Window *f.* Ventana Oval

Overbite *f.* Sobremordida; *f.* Supraoclusión

Oxytone *a.* Agudo-a

P

Pace *m.* Ritmo; *f.* Velocidad; *f.* Rapidez

Palatal *a.* Palatal

Palatal Lift *f.* Prótesis Palatal

Palatalization *f.* Palatalización

Palate *m.* Paladar

Palatoalveolar *a.* Palatoalveolar

Palatoglossal Arch *m.* Arco Palatoglosal

Palatopharyngeal *a.* Palatofaríngeo-a

Palatopharyngeal Arch *m.* Arco Palatofaríngeo

Palatoplasty *f.* Palatoplastia

Palilalia *f.* Palilalia

Palliative Care *m.* Cuidado Paliativo

Paperwork *m.* Papeleo; *m.p* Trámites

Papilloma *m.* Papiloma

Papillomatosis *f.* Papilomatosis

Parahippocampal Gyrus *m.* Giro Parahipocampal

Parallel *a.* Paralelo-a

Paralysis *f.* Parálisis

Paralyzed *a.* Paralizado-a

Paramedic *m/f.* Paramédico-a

Paranoia *f.* Paranoia

Paranoid *a.* Paranoico-a

Paraphasia *f.* Parafasia

Paraplegia *f.* Paraplejía

Paraprofessional *a.* Paraprofesional

Parental *a.* Parental

Parenteral Nutrition *f.* Nutrición Parenteral

Parenting *f.* Crianza

Paresis *f.* Paresia

Parietal Lobe *m.* Lóbulo Parietal

Parkinson's Disease (PD) *f.* Enfermedad de Parkinson

Paroxytone *a.* Llano-a

Pascal *m.* Pascal

Pass Away *v.* Fallecer; *v.* Perder la Vida

Pathological *a.* Patológico-a

Pathologist *m/f.* Patólogo-a

Pathology *f.* Patología

Pathophysiology *f.* Fisiopatología

Pathway *f.* Vía

Patient *m.* Paciente

Patient Chart *f.* Historia Médica del Paciente; Ficha del Paciente

Pause *f.* Pausa

Pedagogical *a.* Pedagógico

Pedagogy *f.* Pedagogía

Pediatric *a.* Pediátrico-a

Peer-Reviewed *a.* Revisado-a por Pares

Penetration *f.* Penetración

Penetration-Aspiration Scale (PAS) *f.* Escala de Penetración-Aspiración (PAS)

Percentage *m.* Porcentaje

Percutaneous Endoscopic Gastrostomy (PEG) *f.* Gastrostomía Endoscópica Percutánea (GEP)

Performative *a.* Performativo

Performative Utterance *f.* Afirmación Performativa; *m.* Enunciado Performativo

Perilymph *f.* Perilinfa

Perinatal *a.* Perinatal

Periodic *a.* Periódico-a

Peripheral *a.* Periférico-a

Peripheral Nervous System (PNS) *m.* Sistema Nervioso Periférico (SNP)

Peristalsis *f.* Peristalsis

Perseveration *f.* Perseverancia

Personality Disorder *m.* Trastorno de Personalidad

Pfeiffer Syndrome *m.* Síndrome de Pfeiffer

Pharmaceutical *a.* Farmacéutico-a

Pharyngeal *a.* Faríngeo-a

Pharyngeal Nerve *m.* Nervio Faríngeo

Pharyngeal Phase *f.* Fase Faríngea

Pharyngealization *f.* Faringealización

Pharyngoesophageal Segment (PES) *m.* Segmento Faringoesofágico; *m.* Esfínter Esofágico Superior (EES)

Pharyngoplasty *f.* Faringoplastia

Pharynogtympanic Tube *m.* Tubo Faringotimpánico; *f.* Trompa Auditiva; *f.* Trompa de Eustaquio; *f.* Tuba

Pharynx *f.* Faringe

Phases of Swallowing *f.p* Etapas de Deglución

Phasic Bite *f.* Mordida Fásica

Phobia *f.* Fobia

Phonation *f.* Fonación

Phoneme *f.* Fonema

Phonemic Awareness *f.* Consciencia Fonémica

Phonemic Transcription *f.* Transcripción Fonémica

Phonestheme *m.* Fonestema

Phonetic *a.* Fonético-a

Phonetic Features *f.p* Características Fonéticas

Phonetic Transcription *f.* Transcripción Fonética

Phonics *m.* Método Silábico

Phonological Alexia *f.* Alexia Fonológica

Phonological Awareness *f.* Consciencia Fonológica

Phonological Processes *m.p* Procesos Fonológicos

Phonology *f.* Fonología

Phonotactics *f.* Fonotáctica

Phrenic Nerve *m.* Nervio Frénico

Physical Therapist *m/f.* Fisioterapeuta

Physical Therapy *f.* Fisioterapia

Physician *m/f.* Doctor-a

Physician's Assistant (PA) *m/f.* Asociado Médico

Physiological *a.* Fisiológico-a

Physiology *f.* Fisiología

Pia Mater *f.* Piamadre

Piaget's Theory of Cognitive Development *f.* Teoría del Desarrollo Cognitivo de Piaget

Pica *f.* Pica; *f.* Enfermedad de Pica

Picture Exchange Communication System (PECS) *m.* Sistema de Comunicación por Intercambio de Imágenes (PECS)

Pidgin *m.* Pidgin

Pinna *m.* Pabellón Auricular

Pitch *m.* Tono

Pituitary Gland *f.* Glándula Pituitaria

Place of Articulation *m.* Punto de Articulación

Platysma Muscle *m.* Músculo Platisma; *m.* Músculo Cutáneo

Play Therapy *f.* Terapia de Juego

Pleura *f.* Pleura

Plosive *f.* Oclusiva; *a.* Oclusivo-a

Pneumonia *f.* Neumonía

Pneumonitis *f.* Neumonitis

Pneumothorax *m.* Neumotórax

Point-of-Care Testing (POCT) *f.p* Pruebas de Laboratorio en el Lugar de Asistencia (POCT)

Pole *m.* Polo

Polyglot *m/f.* Políglota

Polyp *m.* Pólipo

Pons *m.* Puente de Varolio; *m.* Puente Troncoencefálico; *f.* Protuberancia Anular

Portfolio *f.* Carpeta

Positive Reinforcement *m.* Refuerzo Positivo; *m.* Reforzamiento Positivo

Positron Emission Tomography (PET) *f.* Tomografía por Emisión de Positrones (TEP)

Post Mortem *a.* Post Mortem

Postalveolar *a.* Postalveolar; *a.* Prepalatal; *a.* Alveopalatal

Post-Central Gyrus *m.* Giro Poscentral

Posterior *a.* Posterior

Posterior Cerebral Artery (PCA) *f.* Arteria Cerebral Posterior (ACP)

Posterior Horn (Spinal Cord) *m.* Cuerno Posterior (de la Médula Espinal)

Posterior Pharyngeal Flap (PPF) *m.* Colgajo Retrofaríngeo (PPF); *m.* Colgajo Faríngeo (PPF)

Postnatal *a.* Posnatal

Postprandial *a.* Posprandial

Postural *a.* Postural

Posture *f.* Postura

Pragmatics *f.* Pragmática

Precancerous *a.* Precanceroso-a

Precentral Gyrus *m.* Giro Precentral

Precipitating Factor *m.* Factor Desencadenante

Precision *f.* Precisión

Predictive Assessment *f.* Evaluación Predictiva

[111]

Predisposition *f.* Predisposición

Prefix *m.* Prefijo

Prefrontal Cortex (PFC) *f.* Corteza Prefrontal (PFC)

Prelinguistic *a.* Prelingüístico-a; *a.* Prelocutivo-a

Preliteracy *f.* Prealfabetización

Premature *a.* Prematuro-a

Premotor Cortex *f.* Corteza Premotor

Preoperational Stage *f.* Etapa Preoperativa

Presbycusis *f.* Presbiacusia

Presbylaryngis *f.* Presbilaringe

Presbyphagia *f.* Presbiafagia

Preschool *a.* Preescolar

Prescribe *v.* Recetar; *v.* Prescribir

Prescription *f.* Receta

Prescriptive Grammar *m.* Prescriptivismo

Prescriptivist *m/f.* Prescriptivista

Pressure *f.* Presión

Prestige *m.* Prestigio

Preterm *a.* Pretérmino-a

Prevalence *f.* Prevalencia

Prevocalic *a.* Prevocálico -a

Prevoicing *f.* Presonorización

Primary *a.* Primario-a

Primary Progressive Aphasia (PPA) *f.* Afasia Progresiva Primaria (APP); *f.* Afasia de Mesulam

Primary Progressive Apraxia of Speech (PPAOS) *f.* Apraxia Progresiva Primaria del Habla (PPAOS)

Private Practice *f.* Consulta Privada; *f.* Clínica Privada; *m.* Consultorio Privado

Private School *f.* Escuela Privada

Probability *f.* Probabilidad

Probe *f.* Sonda

Problem Solving *f.* Resolución de Problemas

Procedural Memory *f.* Memoria Procedimental

Procedure *m.* Procedimiento

Proficiency *f.* Competencia; *m.* Dominio; *f.* Aptitud

Prognathism *m.* Prognatismo

Prognosis *m.* Pronóstico

Progress *m.* Progreso

Progressive *a.* Progresivo -a

Progressive Assimilation *f.* Asimilación Progresiva

Prone Position *m.* Decúbito Prono; *f.* Posición Prona

Proparoxytone *a.* Esdrújulo-a

Propositional/ Non-Propositional Language *m.* Lenguaje Proposicional/ No Proposicional

Proprioception *f.* Propriocepción

Prosencephalon *m.* Prosencéfalo

Prosodic *a.* Prosódico-a

Prosody *f.* Prosodia

Prosthesis *f.* Prótesis

Prosthetic *a.* Protésico-a

Protein *f.* Proteína

[114]

Prototype *m.* Prototipo

Protrude *v.* Protruir; *v.* Sobresalir

Protrusion *f.* Protrusión

Proxemics *f.* Proxémica

Proximal *a.* Proximal

Psuedobulbar Affect (PBA) *f.* Incontinencia Afectiva

Pseudobulbar Paralysis *f.* Parálisis Pseudobulbar

Pseudoscience *f.* Pseudociencia

Psychiatrist *m/f.* Psiquiatra

Psychiatry *f.* Psiquiatría

Psychogenic *a.* Psicógeno-a

Psycholinguistics *f.* Psicolingüística

Psychological *a.* Psicológico-a

Psychologist *m/f.* Psicólogo-a

Psychology *f.* Psicología

Psychosis *f.* Psicosis

Psychosomatic *a.* Psicosomático-a

[115]

Pterygoid Muscle *m.* Músculo Pterigoideo

Ptosis *f.* Ptosis

Puberty *f.* Pubertad

Pubis *m.* Pubis

Public School *f.* Escuela Pública

Pudding *m.* Pudín

Pulmonary *a.* Pulmonar

Pulmonary Aspiration *f.* Aspiración Pulmonar

Pulmonary Embolism (PE) *f.* Embolia Pulmonar (EP)

Pulmonic *a.* Pulmonar

Puppet *f.* Marioneta; *m.* Muñeco

Puree *m.* Puré

Pure Alexia *f.* Alexia Pura; *f.* Alexia sin Agrafia

Pure Tone Audiometry *f.* Audiometría Tonal

Pure Word Deafness *f.* Sordera Verbal

Purpose *m.* Propósito

Putamen *m.* Putamen

Pyramidal *a*. Piramidal

Pyriform *a*. Piriforme

Q

Quality *f.* Calidad

Quiet Breathing *f.* Respiración Silenciosa; *f.* Respiración Tranquila

Quotient *m.* Cociente

R

Racism *m.* Racismo

Radiation *f.* Radiación

Radiographic *a.* Radiográfico-a

Radiotherapy *f.* Radioterapia

Raised *a.* Elevado-a

Random Sample *f.* Muestra Aleatoria

Range *f.* Gama; *m.* Alcance; *m.* Rango; *m.* Intervalo

Raphe *m.* Rafe

Rare *a.* Raro-a

Rasmussen's Encephalitis (RE) *f.* Encefalitis de Rasmussen (ER)

Rate of Speech *m.* Ritmo del Habla; *f.* Velocidad del Habla

Ratio *f.* Proporción

Receiver in Canal Hearing Aid (RIC) *m.* Audífono con Receptor en el Canal (RIC)

Receptive Aphasia *f.* Afasia Receptiva

Receptive Language *m.* Lenguaje Receptivo

Reciprocity *f.* Reciprocidad

Recognition *m.* Reconocimiento

Recognize *v.* Reconocer

Recovery *f.* Recuperación

Recreational Therapy *f.* Terapia Recreativa

Recurrent Laryngeal Nerve (RLN) *m.* Nervio Laríngeo Recurrente (NLR)

Recurring *a.* Recurrente

Reduction *f.* Reducción

Reduplication *f.* Reduplicación

Refer *v.* Derivar

Reference *f.* Referencia

Referential *a.* Referencial

Referral *f.* Derivación; *m.* Volante (de)

Reflex *m.* Reflejo

Reflux *m.* Reflujo

Reflux Esophagitis *f.* Esofagitis por Reflujo

Register *m.* Registro

Regression *f.* Regresión

Regressive Assimilation *f.* Asimilación Regresiva

Rehabilitation *f.* Rehabilitación

Rehabilitation Center *m.* Centro de Rehabilitación

Reinforcement *m.* Refuerzo; *m.* Reforzamiento

Relevance *f.* Relevancia; *f.* Pertinencia

Remediation *f.* Reparación

Remission *f.* Remisión

Repetition *f.* Repetición

Research *f.* Investigación

Resection *f.* Resección

Residential Care *f.* Atención Residencial; *m.* Cuidado Residencial

Residual *a.* Residual

Residue *m.* Residuo

Resistance *f.* Resistencia

Resonance *f.* Resonancia

Resonant *f.* Sonante; *f.* Sonorante

Resonator *m.* Resonador

Resource Room *m.* Salón de Recursos

Respiration *f.* Respiración

Respiratory Tract *f.p* Vías Respiratorias

Respite Care *f.* Atención de Relevo

Response *f.* Respuesta; *f.* Reacción

Rest Tremor *m.* Temblor de Reposo

Resuscitation *f.* Reanimación; *f.* Resucitación

Reticular Formation (RF) *f.* Formación Reticular (FR)

Retrocochlear *a.* Retrococlear

Retroflex *a.* Retrofleja

Retrograde Amnesia (RA) *f.* Amnesia Retrógrada (AR)

Reversible *a.* Reversible

Rhombencephalon *m.* Rombencéfalo

Rhotacism *m.* Rotacismo

Rhotic *a.* Rótico-a; *f.* Tremulante

Rhyme *f.* Rima

Rhythm *m.* Ritmo

Rib *f.* Costilla

Rib Cage *f.* Caja Torácica

Right Hemisphere Disorder (RHD) *m.* Síndrome del Hemisferio Derecho (RHD); *f.* Lesión del Hemisferio Derecho (RHD)

Risk Factor *m.* Factor de Riesgo

Roof of the Mouth *m.* Paladar; *m.* Techo de la Boca

Rooting Reflex *m.* Reflejo de Búsqueda

Round Window *f.* Ventana Redonda

Rounded *a.* Redondeado-a

Rounding *m.* Redondeamiento

Royal Spanish Academy (RAE) *f.* Real Academia Española (RAE)

Rule *f*. Regla

S

Sacrum *m.* Sacro

Sagittal *a.* Sagital

Salient *a.* Saliente

Saline *a.* Salino-a

Saliva *f.* Saliva

Salivary *a.* Salival

Salivary Gland *f.* Glándula Salival

Sally-Anne Test *f.* Prueba de la Falsa Creencia

Sample *f.* Muestra

Sampling *m.* Muestreo

Saturation *f.* Saturación

Scala Media *f.* Rampa Coclear

Scala Tympani *f.* Rampa Timpánica

Scala Vestibuli *f.* Rampa Vestibular

Scanning *m.* Escaneo

Scanning Speech *f.* Habla Escandida

Scapula *m.* Omóplato; *f.* Escápula

Schatzki's Ring *m.* Anillo de Schatzki; *m.* Anillo Esofágico Inferior

Scheduling *f.* Programación

School Age *a.* (de) Edad Escolar

Schwann Cells *f.p.* Células de Schwann

Scintigraphy *f.* Escintigrafía; *f.* Gammagrafía

Scoliosis *f.* Escoliosis

Screening *m.* Examen; *f.* Prueba; *m.* Cribado

Script *m.* Script

Second Language *f.* Segunda Lengua

Secondary *a.* Secundario-a

Secretion *f.* Secreción

Segment *m.* Segmento

Segmentation *f.* Segmentación

Seizure *f.* Convulsión

Selective Mutism (SM) *m.* Mutismo Selectivo (SM)

Self-Correction *f.* Autocorrección

Self-Help Group *m.* Grupo de Autoayuda

Self-Monitoring *f.* Autocontrol

Self-Regulate *v.* Autorregular

Self-Regulation *f.* Autorregulación

Semantic *a.* Semántico-a

Semantic Alexia *f.* Alexia Semántica

Semantic Feature *m.* Rasgo Semántico

Semantic Feature Analysis *m.* Análisis de Rasgos Semánticos

Semantic Memory *f.* Memoria Semántica

Semantic PPA *f.* APP Semántica

Semantics *f.* Semántica

Semicircular Canals *m.p.* Conductos Semicirculares; *m.p.* Canales Semicirculares

Semiconsonant *f.* Semiconsonante

Semivowel *f.* Semivocal

Senile *a.* Senil

Sensation *f.* Sensación

Sensitive *a.* Sensible

Sensorimotor Stage *f.* Etapa Sensomotora

Sensorineural Hearing Loss *f.* Pérdida Auditiva Sensorineural

Sensory *a.* Sensorial

Sensory Cortex *f.* Corteza Sensorial

Sensory Trick *m.* Gesto Antagonista

Sentence *f.* Frase; *f.* Oración

Sequence *f.* Secuencia

Sequential Swallow *f.* Deglución Secuencial

Serous Membrane *f.* Serosa; *f.* Membrana Serosa

Severe *a.* Severo-a

Sexism *m.* Sexismo

Sexually Transmitted Disease (STD) *f.* Enfermedad de Transmisión Sexual (ETS); *f.* Infección de Transmisión Sexual (ITS)

Shadowing *f.* Observación

Shaping *f.* Modificación

Sheltered *a.* Resguardado-a

Shimmer *m.* Shimmer

Short Vowel *f.* Vocal Corta

Short-Term Memory (STM) *f.* Memoria a Corto Plazo (MCP)

Sibilant *f.* Sibilante ; *a.* Sibilante

Signal-Noise Ratio (SNR) (S/N) *f.* Relación Señal-Ruido (SNR) (S/R)

Sign Language *f.* Lengua de Signos

Signing *v.* Hacer Señas

Silent Aspiration *f.* Aspiración Silenciosa; *f.* Aspiración Callada

Simplification *f.* Simplificación

Singultus *m.* Singulto

Sinus *m.* Seno

Sinusoid *m.* Sinusoide; *a.* Sinusoidal

Skeletal Muscle *m.* Músculo Esquelético

Skilled Nursing Facility (SNF) *m.* Centro de Enfermería Diestro (SNF)

Skull *m.* Cráneo

Sleep Apnea *f.* Apnea del Sueño

Slow Speech *m.* Discurso Lento; *f.* Habla Lenta

Slurred *a.* Mal Articulado-a

Slurring *m.* Mala Articulación

Smooth Muscle *m.* Músculo Liso

Social Skills *f.p.* Habilidades Sociales

Social Worker *m/f.* Asistente Social; *m/f.* Trabajador-a Social

Sociolinguistics *f.* Sociolingüística

Soft Palate *m.* Velo; *m.* Paladar Blando; *m.* Velo del Paladar

Softspoken *a.* De Voz Suave

Soma *m.* Cuerpo Celular

Somatosensory Cortex *f.* Corteza Somatosensorial

Sonorant *f.* Sonante; *f.* Sonorante; *a.* Sonante ; *a.* Sonorante

Sonority *f.* Sonoridad

Sore Throat *m.* Dolor de Garganta; *f.* Garganta Irritada

Sound *m.* Sonido

Source *f.* Fuente

Source-Filter Model *m.* Modelo Fuente-Filtro de la Voz

Spasm *m.* Espasmo

Spasmodic Dysphonia (SD) *f.* Disfonía Espasmódica (SD)

Spastic *a.* Espástico-a

Spastic Dysarthria *f.* Disartria Espástica

Spasticity *f.* Espasticidad

Spatial Awareness *f.* Percepción Espacial

Special Education *f.* Educación Especial; *f.* Educación Diferencial

Specialist *f.* Especialista

Specific Language Impairment (SLI) *m.* Trastorno del Desarrollo del Lenguaje (TDL); *m.* Trastorno Específico del Lenguaje (TEL); *m.* Trastorno Específico del Desarrollo del Lenguaje (TEDL)

Spectrogram *m.* Espectrograma

Spectrum *m.* Espectro

Speech *f.* Habla

Speech Act *m.* Acto de Habla

Speech Apparatus *m.* Aparato Fonador

Speech Audiometry *f.* Logoaudiometría; *f.* Audiometría Verbal

Speech Disorder *m.* Trastorno del Habla

Speech Mechanism *m.* Mecanismo del Habla

Speech Perception *f.* Percepción del Habla

Speech Recognition *m.* Reconocimiento del Habla; *m.* Reconocimiento de Voz

Speech Therapy *f.* Logopedia; *f.* Terapia del Habla; *f.* Terapia del Lenguaje

Speech-Language Pathologist (SLP) *m/f.* Patólogo-a del Habla y Lenguaje; *m/f.* Logopeda; *m/f.* Terapeuta del Habla; *m/f.* Fonoaudiólogo

Speech-Language Pathology *f.* Logopedia; *f.* Patología del Habla y Lenguaje; *f.* Fonoaudiología

Speech-Language Pathology Assistant (SLPA) *m.* Auxiliar al Patólogo del Habla y Lenguaje (SLPA)

Sphincter *m.* Esfínter

Spillage *m.* Derrame

Spina Bifida *f.* Espina Bífida

Spinal Cord *f.* Médula Espinal

Spinal Cord Injury (SCI) *f.* Lesión de la Médula Espinal (LME)

Spinal Ganglia *m.p.* Ganglios Espinales; *m.p.* Ganglios de las Raíces Dorsales

Spirant *f.* Espirante; *a.* Espirante

Spirantization *f.* Espirantización

[133]

Split-Brain *m*. Cerebro Dividido

Spondee *m*. Espondeo

Spontaneous *a*. Espontáneo-a

Standard Deviation *f*. Desviación Típica; *f*. Desviación Estándar

Standardized *a*. Estandarizado-a

Stapedius *m*. Músculo Estapedio; *m*. Músculo del Estribo

Stapes *m*. Estribo

Statistic *f*. Estadística

Statistically Significant *a*. Estadísticamente Significativo-a

Status *m*. Estado

Steadiness *f*. Firmeza; *f*. Estabilidad

Steady Pace *m*. Ritmo Estable; *m*. Ritmo Constante

Stem Cells *f.p*. Células Madre; *f.p*. Células Troncales

Stenosis *m*. Estenosis

Stereocilia *f*. Estereocilia

Sternum *m*. Esternón

Stethoscope *m.* Estetoscopio

Stigma *m.* Estigma

Stigmatized *a.* Estigmatizado-a

Stimulus *m.* Estímulo

Stoma *f.* Estoma

Stop *f.* Oclusiva

Stopping *f.* Oclusivización

Strategy *f.* Estrategia

Stress *m.* Acento; *m.* Acento Tónico; *m.* Énfasis; *m.* Acento Prosódico

Stressed *a.* Tónico-a

Striated Muscle *m.* Músculo Estriado

Striatum *m.* Cuerpo Estriado; *m.* Núcleo Estriado

Strident *m.* Estridente

Stridor *m.* Estridor

Strobosocopy *f.* Estroboscopia

Stroke *m.* Ictus; *m.* Accidente Cerebrovascular (ACV); *f.* Apoplejía; *f.* Enfermedad Cerebrovascular; *m.* Infarto Cerebral

Stutter *v.* Tartamudear

Stuttering *f.* Tartamudez

Subacute *a.* Subagudo-a

Subarachnoid *a.* Subaracnoideo-a

Subdural *a.* Subdural

Subglottal *a.* Subglótico-a

Substantia Nigra *f.* Sustancia Negra

Substitute *v.* Sustituir

Substitution *f.* Sustitución

Subthalamus *m.* Subtálamo

Successive *a.* Sucesivo-a; *a.* Consecutivo-a; *a.* Seguido-a

Sucking Reflex *m.* Reflejo de Succión

Suckling *f.* Lactación

Sudden Infant Death Syndrome (SIDS) *m.* Síndrome de Muerte Súbita del Lactante (SMSL)

Suffix *m.* Sufijo

Sulcus *m.* Surco

Summative Assessment *f.* Evaluación Sumativa

Superficial *a.* Superficial

Superior *a.* Superior

Superior Canal Dehiscence Syndrome (SCDS) *m.* Síndrome de Dehiscencia del Canal Superior (SCDS)

Superior Laryngeal Nerve (SLN) *m.* Nervio Laríngeo Superior (NLS)

Superior Olivary Complex (SOC) *m.* Complejo Olivar Superior (COS); *m.* Núcleo Olivar Superior (NOS)

Supine Position *m.* Decúbito Supino; *f.* Posición Supina

Support Group *m.* Grupo de Apoyo

Supracricoid *a.* Supracricoideo

Supraglottal *a.* Supraglótico-a

Suprahyoid Muscles *m.p* Músculos Suprahioideos

Supramarginal Gyrus *m.* Giro Supramarginal

Surface Alexia *f.* Alexia de Superficie

[137]

Suture *f.* Sutura

Swallowing *f.* Deglución

Swallowing Disorder *m.* Trastorno de Deglución

Swallowing Therapy *m.* Tratamiento de la Deglución; *m.* Tratamiento Para la Disfagia

Swelling *f.* Hinchazón; *f.* Inflamación

Swollen *a.* Hinchado-a; *a.* Inflamado-a

Syllabification *f.* Silabificación

Syllable *f.* Sílaba

Sylvian Fissure *f.* Cisura de Silvio; *m.* Surco Lateral

Symbolic Play *m.* Juego Simbólico

Sympathetic Nervous System *m.* Sistema Nervioso Simpático

Symphysis *f.* Sínfisis

Symptom *m.* Síntoma

Synalepha *f.* Sinalefa

Synapse *f.* Sinapsis

Synaptic *a.* Sináptico-a

Synaptic Pruning *f.* Poda Sináptica; *f.* Poda Neuronal

Synaptogenesis *f.* Sinaptogénesis

Syndrome *m.* Síndrome

Syntax *f.* Sintaxis

Synthesis *f.* Síntesis

S/Z Ratio *f.* Relación S/Z

T

Tachycardia *f*. Taquicardia

Tactile *a*. Táctil

Tap *f*. Vibrante Simple

Tardive Dyskinesia (TD) *f*. Discinesia Tardía (TD)

Target *m*. Objetivo; *f*. Meta

Tau Protein *f*. Proteína Tau

Team *m*. Equipo

Tear *m*. Desgarro

Teeth *m.p*. Dientes

Telegraphic Speech *f*. Habla Telegráfica

Telencephalon *m*. Telencéfalo

Telepractice *f*. Telepráctica

Teletherapy *f*. Teleterapia

Temporal Lobe *m*. Lóbulo Temporal

Tense Vowel *f*. Vocal Tensa

Tension *m.* Tensión

Tensor Tympani *m.* Músculo Tensor del Tímpano; *m.* Músculo del Martillo

Teratogenesis *f.* Teratogénesis

Test *f.* Prueba; *m.* Examen

Test Battery *f.* Batería de Pruebas

Thalamic *a.* Talámico-a

Thalamic Pain Syndrome *m.* Síndrome Talámico; *m.* Síndrome de Dejerine–Roussy

Thalamus *m.* Tálamo

Theory *f.* Teoría

Theory of Mind *f.* Teoría de la Mente

Therapy *f.* Terapia; *m.* Tratamiento

Thin Liquid *m.* Líquido Fino; *m.* Líquido Claro

Thoracic *a.* Torácico

Thoracic Cage *f.* Caja Torácica

Threshold *m.* Umbral

Thrombectomy *f.* Trombectomía

Thrombosis *f.* Trombosis

Thrombotic Stroke *m.* Ictus Trombótico

Thrombus *m.* Trombo

Thyroid *f.* Tiroides

Thyroid Cartilage *m.* Cartílago Tiroides

Thyroid Gland *f.* Glándula Tiroides

Thyroplasty *f.* Tiroplastia

Tic *m.* Tic

Tinnitus *m.p.* Tinnitus; *m.p.* Acúfenos

Tissue *m.* Tejido

Tissue Plasminogen Activator (tPA) *m.* Activador Tisular del Plasminógeno (t-PA)

Tongue *f.* Lengua

Tongue Depressor *m.* Depresor Lingual

Tongue Thrust *m.* Empuje de la Lengua

Tonotopic *a.* Tonotópico-a

Tonsil *f.* Amígdala

Tonsilectomy *f.* Amigdalectomía

Tonsillitis *f.* Tonsilitis

Torticollis *f.* Tortícolis

Total Communication (TC) *f.* Comunicación Total (TC)

Total Parenteral Nutrition (TPN) *f.* Nutrición Parenteral Total (NPT)

Total Physical Response (TPR) *f.* Respuesta Física Total (TPR)

Tourette Syndrome (TS) *m.* Síndrome de Tourette (TS)

Trachea *f.* Tráquea

Tracheoesophageal *a.* Traqueoesofágico-a

Tracheoesophageal Fistula *f.* Fístula Traqueoesofágica

Tracheomalacia *f.* Traqueomalacia

Tracheostomy *f.* Traqueostomía

Tracheotomy *f.* Traqueotomía

Tract *m.* Tracto; *m.* Aparato

Transcortical Aphasia *f.* Afasia Transcortical

Transcortical Motor Aphasia (TMA) *f.* Afasia Transcortical Motora (ATM)

Transcortical Sensory Aphasia (TSA) *f.* Afasia Transcortical Sensorial (ATS)

Transcription *f.* Transcripción

Transformational Grammar *f.* Gramática Generativa Transformacional

Transgender *a.* Transgénero; *a.* Transexual

Transglottal *a.* Transglótico-a

Transient *a.* Transitorio-a

Transient Ischemic Attack (TIA) *m.* Accidente Isquémico Transitorio (AIT)

Transitional *a.* Transitorio-a

Translate *v.* Traducir

Translation *f.* Traducción

Transneuronal Degeneration *f.* Degeneración Transneuronal

Transverse *a.* Transversal

Trapezius *m.* Trapecio

Trauma *m.* Trauma

Traumatic *a.* Traumático-a

Traumatic Brain Injury (TBI) *f.* Lesión Cerebral Traumática (LCT)

Travel Therapy *f.* Terapia del Viaje

Treatment *m.* Tratamiento

Tremor *m.* Temblor

Triage *m.* Triaje

Triangular Part *f.* Parte Triangular

Trigeminal Nerve *m.* Nervio Trigémino

Trigraph *m.* Trígrafo

Trilingual *a.* Trilingüe

Trill *f.* Vibrante Múltiple

Triphthong *m.* Triptongo

Trisomy *f.* Trisomía

Trochlear Nerve *m*. Nervio Troclear; *m*. Nervio Patético

Tube *f*. Sonda; *m*. Tubo

Tumor *m*. Tumor

Turn Taking *v*. Tomar Turnos

Tympanic Duct *f*. Rampa Timpánica

Tympanic Membrane *f*. Membrana Timpánica; *m*. Tímpano; *f*. Caja Timpánica

Tympanometry *f*. Timpanometría

Type *m*. Tipo; *m*. Grupo

U

Ulcer *f.* Úlcera

Ultrasound *m.* Ultrasonido

Unaided Communication *f.* Comunicación Sin Ayuda

Underbite *f.* Submordida

Unilateral *a.* Unilateral

Unilateral Vocal Cord Paralysis *f.* Parálisis Unilateral de las Cuerdas Vocales

University *f.* Universidad

Unmarked *a.* No Marcado

Unrounded *a.* No Redondeada

Unstressed *a.* Átono-a

Upper *a.* Superior

Upper Esophageal Sphincter (UES) *m.* Esfínter Esofágico Superior (EES)

Upper Motor Neuron (UMN) *f.* Neurona Motora Superior (NMS)

Utterance *f.* Expresión; *f.* Declaración; *f.* Afirmación; *m.* Enunciado

Uvula *f.* Úvula

Uvular *a.* Uvular

V

Vaccination *f.* Vacunación

Vaccine *f.* Vacuna

Vagotomy *f.* Vagotomía

Vagus Nerve *m.* Nervio Vago; *m.* Nervio Neumogástrico

Validity *f.* Validez

Vallecula *f.* Vallécula

Valve *f.* Válvula

Variability *f.* Variabilidad

Variable *f.* Variable

Vascular *a.* Vascular

Vasovagal *a.* Vasovagal

Vein *f.* Vena

Velar *a.* Velar

Velarization *f.* Velarización

Velocardiofacial Syndrome (VCFS) *m.* Síndrome Velocardiofacial (VCFS)

Velopharyngeal *a.* Velofaríngeo-a

Velopharyngeal Closure *m.* Cierre Velofaríngeo

Velopharyngeal Insufficiency (VPI) *f.* Insuficiencia Velofaríngea (IVF)

Velopharyngeal Port (VPP) *m.* Puerto Velofaríngeo (PVF); Mecanismo Velofaríngeo (MV)

Velum *m.* Velo

Ventral *a.* Ventral

Ventricle *m.* Ventrículo

Ventricular *a.* Ventricular

Verbal *a.* Verbal

Verbal Apraxia *f.* Apraxia Verbal

Verbal Communication *f.* Comunicación Verbal

Vernacular *a.* Vernáculo-a

Vertebra *f.* Vértebra

Vertebrobasilar Insufficiency (VBI) *f.* Insuficiencia Vertebrobasilar (IVB)

Vertigo *m.* Vértigo

Vestibular Duct *f.* Rampa Vestibular

Vestibular Fold *m.* Pliegue Vestibular

Vestibular Nerve *m.* Nervio Vestibular

Vestibular Schwannoma *f.* Schwanoma Vestibular; *f.* Neurinoma Vestibular; *f.* Neurinoma del Acústico

Vestibule *m.* Vestíbulo

Vestibulocochlear Nerve *m.* Nervio Vestibulococlear; *m.* Nervio Estatoacústico; *m.* Nervio Auditivo

Veteran *m/f.* Veterano-a

Veteran's Affairs *m.p.* Asuntos de Veteranos

Vibrate *v.* Vibrar

Vibration *f.* Vibración

Videofluoroscopic *a.* Video Fluoroscópico-a

Visceral *a.* Visceral

Viscosity *f.* Viscosidad

Viscous *a.* Viscoso-a

Viseme *m.* Viseme

Visual Agnosia *f.* Agnosia Visual

Visual Motor *a.* Visomotriz

Visual Word Form Area (VWFA) *m.* Área Visual de Formación de Palabras (VWFA)

Vocabulary *m.* Vocabulario

Vocal Cords *f.p* Cuerdas Vocales

Vocal Fatigue *f.* Fatiga Vocal

Vocal Fold *m.* Pliegue Vocal

Vocal Fry *m.* Registro Glotal; *m.* Registro Laríngeo

Vocal Intensity *f.* Intensidad Vocal

Vocal Strain *m.* Esfuerzo Vocal

Vocal Tension *f.* Tensión Vocal

Vocal Tract *m.* Tracto Vocal

Vocal Tremor *m.* Temblor Vocal

Vocalization *f.* Vocalización

Vocoid *m.* Vocoide

Voice *f.* Voz

Voice Box *f.* Laringe

Voice Coach *m/f.* Profesor-a de Voz

Voice Disorder *m.* Trastorno de la Voz

Voiced *a.* Sonoro-a

Voiceless *a.* Sordo-a; *a.* Insonoro-a

Voicing *f.* Sonoridad; *f.* Sonorización

Volitional *a.* Volitivo-a

Voltage *f.* Tensión; *m.* Voltaje

Volume *m.* Volumen

Voluntary *a.* Voluntario-a

Vowel *f.* Vocal

W

Wada Test *m*. Test de Wada; *f*. Prueba de Wada

Wallerian Degeneration *f*. Degeneración Walleriana

Wave *f*. Onda

Wavelength *f*. Longitud de Onda

Weak Syllable Deletion *f*. Supresión de Sílabas Átonas

Wernicke's Aphasia *f*. Afasia de Wernicke

Wernicke's Area *m*. Área de Wernicke

White Matter *f*. Sustancia Blanca

Williams Syndrome (WS) *m*. Síndrome de Williams (WS)

Withing Normal Limits (WNL) *a*. Dentro de Límites Normales (DLN)

Word Association *f*. Asociación de Palabras

Word Finding *f*. Evocación de Palabras

Working Memory *f*. Memoria de Trabajo

X

X-Ray *f.* Radiografía; *m.p* Rayos X

Y

Youth *f*. Juventud

Z

Zenker's Diverticulum *m.* Divertículo de Zenker

Zone of Proximal Development (ZPD) *f.* Zona de Desarrollo Próximo (ZDP)

Zygomatic Arch *m.* Arco Cigomático

Guía Para los Términos Español-Inglés

Este libro ofrece una lista integral de términos que son comunes a los estudios de lenguaje, habla, y audición, especialmente la fonoaudiología, pero también incluye términos relevantes para la audiología, la lingüística, la neurología y la pedagogía. Cabe decir que ninguna referencia única realmente puede contener toda la terminología y jerga que existe en estos dominios. Sin embargo, este libro intenta cubrir las selecciones de palabras más importantes que son relevantes para muchos tipos de fonoaudiólogos en una variedad de entornos. El propósito de este libro es servir como referencia de traducción, ayudando en el desarrollo de habilidades bilingües relevantes para el campo y cerrando la brecha entre fonoaudiólogos de diferentes orígenes.

Los nombres y abreviaturas de evaluaciones estandarizadas, como la CLQT+, no se incluyen en este glosario ni en sus apéndices. Sin embargo, en este libro se mencionan muchos procedimientos que se utilizan ampliamente, que no se consideran evaluaciones estandarizadas.

Las palabras y frases en español se enumeran en orden alfabético según la primera letra de la palabra o la primera palabra de la frase. Las traducciones en inglés no están ordenadas alfabéticamente para esta sección ya que están correlacionadas con los términos en español. Todas las palabras significativas de los términos en inglés y español se escriben con mayúscula para mantener la coherencia.

La palabra o frase en español que se traduce está impresa en **negrita**.

La palabra o frase va seguida de una letra en *cursiva* que indica la parte gramatical de la traducción. Para las traducciones al inglés, las abreviaturas de la parte gramatical incluyen *n.* (sustantivo), *a.* (adjetivo) y *v.* (verbo). Cuando una palabra es plural en la traducción dada, una *p.* seguirá la parte gramatical.

La traducción al inglés de la palabra sigue la parte gramatical y está impresa en texto sin formato.

Los adjetivos en español se escriben en forma masculina. Tanto los verbos en inglés como sus traducciones al español se presentan en la forma infinitiva del verbo, excepto cuando un término específico casi siempre se encuentra en una forma diferente.

Las frases que tienen abreviaturas comunes tendrán la abreviatura entre paréntesis al final de la frase. La frase traducida también incluirá la abreviatura más utilizada en el idioma opuesto. En algunos casos, la abreviatura puede ser diferente en inglés que en español, cuando el español tiene su propia abreviatura para una frase, pero en otros casos la abreviatura permanecerá igual cuando el español usa las siglas del inglés. Consulte el Apéndice I para consultar rápidamente una lista de abreviaturas seleccionadas en inglés, o el Apéndice II para abreviaturas en español.

Cuando una frase tiene más de una traducción común, las traducciones están separadas por punto y coma. Cada nueva traducción irá precedida de su propia parte gramatical.

Algunas palabras pueden aparecer varias veces en diferentes contextos o como parte de otras frases. Otras palabras pueden aparecer en diferentes formas o diferentes partes gramaticales como frases separadas, cuando la diferencia entre las dos es significativa en la traducción o cuando ambas versiones se utilizan con frecuencia. Algunos sustantivos y adjetivos pueden aparecer como frases separadas, así como en una frase combinada, cuando proceda. En primer lugar aparecerá la traducción preferida o más utilizada, seguida de sus otras posibles variaciones.

[161]

La sección que sigue es la colección de traducciones inglés-español. Para los términos español-inglés, consulte la página 10.

A

Abdomen *n.* Abdomen

Abdominal *a.* Abdominal

Abducción *n.* Abduction

Abducir *v.* Abduct

Abecedario *n.* Alphabet; *n.p.* ABCs

Abertura *n.* Opening; *n.* Aperture

Ablación *n.* Ablation

Abogar *v.* Advocate

Abstracción *n.* Abstraction

Abulia *n.* Aboulia

Abuso *n.* Abuse

Abuso Infantil *n.* Child Abuse

Acalasia *n.* Achalasia

Acalculia *n.* Acalculia

Accesibilidad *n.* Accessibility

Accidente Cerebrovascular (ACV) *n.* Cerebrovascular Accident (CVA); *n.* Stroke

Accidente de Vehículo de Motor (AVM) *n.* Motor Vehicle Accident (MVA)

Accidente Isquémico Transitorio (AIT) *n.* Transient Ischemic Attack (TIA)

Acento *n.* Accent

Acento Tónico *n.* Stress

Acidez *n.* Heartburn

Ácido Desoxirribonucleico (ADN) *n.* Deoxyribonucleic Acid (DNA)

Ácido Gamma-Aminobutírico (GABA) *n.* Gamma-Aminobutyric Acid

Acinesia *n.* Akinesia

Acinético *a.* Akinetic

Acreditado *a.* Accredited; *a.* Certified

Activador Tisular del Plasminógeno (t-PA) *n.* Tissue Plasminogen Activator (tPA)

Actividades de la Vida Diaria (ACVD) *n.p.* Activities of Daily Living (ADL)

Acto de Habla *n.* Speech Act

Acúfenos *n.* Tinnitus

Aculturación *n.* Acculturation

Acústico *a.* Acoustic

Adaptación *n.* Adaptation

Administración de Alimentos y Medicamentos (FDA) *n.* Food and Drug Administration (FDA)

Adolescente *a.* Adolescent

Adquisición *n.* Acquisition

Aducción *n.* Adduction

Aducción Aritenoidea *n.* Arytenoid Adduction

Aducir *v.* Adduct

Adulto *a.* Adult

Aerodigestivo *a.* Aerodigestive

Afasia *n.* Aphasia

Afasia Anómica *n*. Anomic Aphasia

Afasia de Mesulam *n*. Primary Progressive Aphasia (PPA)

Afasia Dinámica *n*. Dynamic Aphasia

Afasia Expresiva *n*. Expressive Aphasia

Afasia Fluente *n*. Fluent Aphasia

Afasia Global *n*. Global Aphasia

Afasia No Fluente *n*. Nonfluent Aphasia

Afasia Progresiva Primaria (APP) *n*. Primary Progressive Aphasia (PPA)

Afasia Receptiva *n*. Receptive Aphasia

Afasia Transcortical *n*. Transcortical Aphasia

Afasia Transcortical Mixta *n*. Mixed Transcortical Aphasia (MTA/MTCA)

Afasia Transcortical Motora (ATM) *n*. Transcortical Motor Aphasia (TMA)

Afasia Transcortical Sensorial (ATS) *n*. Transcortical Sensory Aphasia (TSA)

Afasia de Broca *n*. Broca's Aphasia

Afasia de Conducción *n.* Conduction Aphasia

Afasia de Wernicke *n.* Wernicke's Aphasia

Afásico *a.* Aphasic

Aferente *a.* Afferent

Afijo *n.* Affix

Afonía *n.* Aphonia

Africada *n.* Affricate; *a.* Affricate

Agnosia *n.* Agnosia

Agnosia Digital *n.* Finger Agnosia

Agnosia Visual *n.* Visual Agnosia

Agrafia Agraphia

Agramatismo *n.* Agrammatism

Agudo *a.* Acute; *a.* Oxytone

Agujero Magno *n.* Foramen Magnum

Aislamiento *n.* Isolation

Alalia *n.* Alalia

Alcance *n.* Scope; *n.* Reach; *n.* Range

Alergia *n.* Allergy

Alérgico *a.* Allergic

Alexia *n.* Alexia

Alexia de Superficie *n.* Surface Alexia

Alexia Fonológica *n.* Phonological Alexia

Alexia Profunda *n.* Deep Alexia

Alexia Pura *n.* Pure Alexia; *n.* Alexia Without Agraphia

Alexia Semántica *n.* Semantic Alexia

Alfabetización *n.* Literacy

Alfabetización en Salud *n.* Health Literacy

Alfabetizado *a.* Literate

Alfabeto *n.* Alphabet

Alfabeto Fonético Internacional (AFI) *n.* International Phonetic Alphabet (IPA)

Alfabeto Manual *n.* Fingerspelling; *n.* Manual Alphabet

Alimentación *n.* Feeding

Alimentación Nasogástrica *n*. Nasogastric Feeding

Alimentario *a*. Alimentary; *a*. Dietary

Alimenticio *a*. Dietary; *a*. Alimentary

Alófono *n*. Allophone

Alternancia de Código *n*. Code-Switching

Alucinación *n*. Hallucination

Alveolar *a*. Alveolar

Alvéolos *n.p*. Alveoli; *n*. Alveolar Ridge

Alveopalatal *a*. Alveopalatal

Ambiente Menos Restrictivo *n*. Least Restrictive Environment

Ambulatorio *a*. Outpatient; *a*. Ambulatory

Amígdala *n*. Tonsil

Amigdalectomía *n*. Tonsilectomy

Amnesia *n*. Amnesia

Amnesia Anterógrada (AA) *n*. Anterograde Amnesia (AA)

Amnesia Retrógrada (AR) *n*. Retrograde Amnesia (RA)

[169]

Amplificación *n*. Amplification

Amplitud *n*. Amplitude

Anafilaxia *n*. Anaphylaxis

Analfabetismo *n*. Illiteracy

Analfabeto *a*. Illiterate

Análisis *n*. Analysis

Análisis del Comportamiento Aplicado (ABA) *n*. Applied Behavior Analysis (ABA)

Analista del Comportamiento Acreditado (BCBA) *n*. Board Certified Behavior Analyst (BCBA)

Análisis de Rasgos Semánticos *n*. Semantic Feature Analysis

Anartria *n*. Anarthria

Anastomosis *n*. Anastomosis

Anatomía *n*. Anatomy

Andadura *n*. Gait

Anencefalia *n*. Anencephaly

Anestesia *n.* Anesthesia

Anestesiólogo *n.* Anesthesiologist

Aneurisma *n.* Aneurism

Angiografía *n.* Angiography

Anillo Esofágico *n.* Esophageal Ring

Anillo de Schatzki *n.* Schatzki's Ring

Anomalía *n.* Anomaly

Anomalías Craneofaciales *n.p.* Craniofacial Anomalies

Anomia *n.* Anomia

Anopsia *n.* Anopsia

Anorexia *n.* Anorexia

Anormalidad *n.* Abnormality

Anotia *n.* Anotia

Anoxia *n.* Anoxia

Anquiloglosia *n.* Ankyloglossia

Anterior *n.* Anterior

Anterioridad *n.* Frontedness

Anteriorización *n.* Fronting

Anteriorizado *a.* Fronted

Antropología *n.* Anthropology

Aorta *n.* Aorta

Aparato Fonador *n.p.* Organs of Speech; *n.* Speech Apparatus

Aparición Tardía del Lenguaje (LLE) *n.* Late Language Emergence (LLE)

Apendicular *a.* Appendicular

Apical *a.* Apical

Ápice *n.* Apex

Apnea de Sueño *n.* Sleep Apnea

Apoplejía *n.* Stroke; *n.* Apoplexy

Apoptosis *n.* Apoptosis

APP Agramática *n.* Agrammatic PPA; Nonfluent PPA

APP Logopénica *n.* Logopenic PPA

APP Semántica *n*. Semantic PPA

Apraxia *n*. Apraxia

Apraxia Bucofacial *n*. Buccofacial Apraxia

Apraxia Conceptual *n*. Conceptual Apraxia

Apraxia Constructiva *n*. Constructional Apraxia

Apraxia del Vestir *n*. Dressing Apraxia

Apraxia Ideomotora *n*. Ideomotor Apraxia

Apraxia Motriz *n*. Motor Apraxia

Apraxia Verbal *n*. Verbal Apraxia

Apraxia de Extremidad Cinética *n*. Limb-Kinetic Apraxia

Apraxia de la Marcha *n*. Gait Apraxia

Apraxia del Habla (AOS) *n*. Apraxia of Speech (AOS)

Apraxia del Habla Infantil (CAS) *n*. Childhood Apraxia of Speech (CAS)

Apraxia Progresiva Primaria del Habla (PPAOS) *n*. Primary Progressive Apraxia of Speech (PPAOS)

Aprendizaje *n*. Learning

Aprendizaje Motor *n.* Motor Learning

Aprosodia *n.* Aprosodia

Aproximante *n.* Approximant; *a.* Approximant

Aptitud *n.* Aptitude; *n.* Ability; *n.* Proficiency

Aracnoides *n.* Arachnoid Mater

Arco Cigomático *n.* Zygomatic Arch

Arco Dental *n.* Dental Arch

Arco Palatofaríngeo *n.* Palatopharyngeal Arch

Arco Palatoglosal *n.* Palatoglossal Arch

Arcos Fauciales *n.p.* Faucial Arches

Área de Broca *n.* Broca's Area

Área de Wernicke *n.* Wernicke's Area

Área Visual de Formación de Palabras (VWFA) *n.* Visual Word Form Area (VWFA)

Áreas de Brodmann *n.p.* Brodmann Areas

Ariepiglotal *a.* Aryepiglottal

Aritenoides *n.* Arytenoids

Arousal Cortical *n.* Cortical Arousal

Arrullar *v.* Coo

Arrullo *n.* Cooing

Arteria *n.* Artery

Arteria Basilar *n.* Basilar Artery

Arteria Carótida Común *n.* Common Carotid Artery

Arteria Cerebral Anterior (ACA) *n.* Anterior Cerebral Artery (ACA)

Arteria Cerebral Media (ACM) *n.* Middle Cerebral Artery

Arteria Cerebral Posterior (ACP) *n.* Posterior Cerebral Artery

Arteria Comunicante *n.* Communicating Artery

Articulación *n.* Articulation; *n.* Joint

Articulación a Tientas *n.* Articulatory Groping

Articuladores *n.* Articulators

Artritis *n.* Arthritis

Asemia *n.* Asemia

Asesor *n.* Advisor; *n.* Counselor

Asesoramiento *n.* Counseling

Asfixia *n.* Asphyxia ; *n.* Asphyxiation

Asibilación *n.* Assibilation

Asimetría *n.* Asymmetry

Asimétrico *a.* Asymmetrical

Asimilación *n.* Assimilation

Asimilación Progresiva *n.* Progressive Assimilation

Asimilación Regresiva *n.* Regressive Assimilation

Asintomático *a.* Asymptomatic

Asistente Social *n.* Social Worker

Asistente Certificado de Terapia Ocupacional (COTA) *n.* Certified Occupational Therapy Assistant (COTA)

Asma *n.* Asthma

Asmático *a.* Asthmatic

Asociación Americana de Habla, Lenguaje y Audición (ASHA) *n.* American Speech-Language-Hearing Association (ASHA)

Asociación Nacional para la Educación Bilingüe (NABE) *n.* National Association for Bilingual Education (NABE)

Asociación de Palabras *n.* Word Association

Asociado Médico *n.* Physician's Assistant (PA)

Aspectos Lingüísticos *n.p.* Linguistic Aspects

Aspiración *n.* Aspiration

Aspiración Pulmonar *n.* Pulmonary Aspiration

Aspiración Silenciosa *n.* Silent Aspiration

Aspirado *a.* Aspirated

Aspirar *v.* Aspirate

Astrocito *n.* Astrocyte

Asuntos de Veteranos *n.p.* Veteran's Affairs

Ataque *n.* Onset; *n.* Attack

Ataxia *n.* Ataxia

Ataxia de Freidreich *n.* Freidreich's Ataxia

Atáxico *a.* Ataxic

Atención Médica Domiciliaria *n.* Home Health Care

Atención a Largo Plazo *n.* Long-Term Treatment; *n.* Long-Term Care

Atención de Agudos *n.* Acute Care

Atención de Revelo *n.* Respite Care

Atenuación *n.* Attenuation

Atestiguado *a.* Attested

Atetosis *n.* Athetosis

Atresia *n.* Atresia

Atresia Coanal *n.* Choanal Atresia

Atresia Esofágica *n.* Esophageal Atresia

Atrofia *n.* Atrophy

Atrofia Olivopontocerebelosa (OPCA) *n.* Olivopontocerebellar Atrophy (OPCA)

Átono *a.* Unstressed

Audición *n.* Hearing; *n.* Audition

Audífono *n.* Hearing Aid

Audífono Completamente en el Canal (CIC) *n.* Completely in Canal Hearing Aid (CIC)

Audífono con Anclaje Óseo (BAHA) *n.* Bone-Anchored Hearing Aid (BAHA); *n.* Bone-Anchored Hearing Implant (BAHI)

Audífono con Receptor en el Canal (RIC) *n.* Receiver in Canal Hearing Aid (RIC)

Audífono Intrauricular (ITE) *n.* In the Ear Hearing Aid (ITE)

Audífono Retroauricular (BTE) *n.* Behind the Ear Hearing Aid (BTE)

Audiograma *n.* Audiogram

Audiología *n.* Audiology

Audiólogo *n.* Audiologist

Audiometría *n.* Audiometry

Audiometría Tonal *n.* Pure Tone Audiometry

Audiometría Verbal *n.* Speech Audiometry

Audiómetro *n.* Audiometer

Aumento *n.* Augmentation

Auscultación *n.* Auscultation

Auscultación Cervical *n.* Cervical Auscultation

Autismo *n.* Autism

Autocontrol *n.* Self-Control; *n.* Self-Monitoring

Autocorrección *n.* Self-Correction

Autopsia *n.* Autopsy

Autorregulación *n.* Self-Regulation

Autorregular *v.* Self-Regulate

Axial *a.* Axial

Axón *n.* Axon

B

Balbucear *v*. Babble

Balbuceo *n*. Babbling

Balbuceo Marginal *n*. Marginal Babbling

Barbarismo *n*. Barbarism

Barbilla Hacia Abajo *n*. Chin Tuck; *n*. Chin Down

Bario *n*. Barium

Barrera Hematoencefálica (BHE) *n*. Blood-Brain Barrier (BBB)

Barreras Lingüísticas *n.p.* Linguistic Barriers; *n.p.* Language Barriers

Barreras de Acceso *n.p.* Access Barriers

Base *n*. Base; *n*. Baseline

Base de la Boca *n*. Floor of the Mouth

Batería de Pruebas *n*. Test Battery

Becario Clínico *n*. Clinical Fellow

Benigno *a*. Benign

Bilabial *a.* Bilabial

Bilateral *a.* Bilateral

Bilingüe *a.* Bilingual

Bilingüismo *n.* Bilingualism

Bilirrubina *n.* Bilirubin

Binaural *a.* Binaural

Biopsia *n.* Biopsy

Biopsicosocial *n.* Biopsychosocial

Bolo *n.* Bolus

Bradicinesia *n.* Bradykinesia

Bronquiolos *n.p.* Bronchioles

Bronquios *n.p.* Bronchi

Bucal *a.* Buccal

Bulbar *a.* Bulbar

Bulbo Olfativo *n.* Olfactory Bulb

Bulbo Raquídeo *n.* Medulla Oblongata

C

Cadena Osicular *n.* Ossicular Chain

Caja Torácica *n.* Thoracic Cage; *n.* Rib Cage

Calibrar *v.* Calibrate

Calidad *n.* Quality

Cambio de Código *n.* Code-Switching

Campo Ocular Frontal *n.* Frontal Eye Field

Cáncer *n.* Cancer

Cáncer de Cabeza y Cuello *n.* Head and Neck Cancer

Canceroso *a.* Cancerous

Candidatura *n.* Candidacy

Cánula *n.* Cannula

Capacidad de Atención *n.* Attention

Cápsula Interna *n.* Internal Capsule

Caracol *n.* Cochlea

Características Fonéticas *n.p.* Phonetic Features

[183]

Cardíaco *a.* Cardiac

Carga de Trabajo *n.* Workload; *n.* Caseload

Carpeta *n.* Portfolio; *n.* File

Cartílago *n.* Cartilage

Cartílago Cricoides *n.* Cricoid Cartilage

Cartílago Tiroides *n.* Thyroid Cartilage

Catarro *n.* Cold

Catéter *n.* Catheter

Cavidad *n.* Cavity

Cavidad Bucal *n.* Buccal Cavity

Cavidad Nasal *n.* Nasal Cavity

Cavidad Oral *n.* Oral Cavity

Ceceo *n.* Lisp

Células Ciliadas *n.p.* Hair Cells

Células de Schwann *n.p.* Schwann Cells

Células Gliales *n.p.* Glial Cells

Células Madre *n.p.* Stem Cells

Ceguera *n.* Blindness

Ceguera Cortical *n.* Cortical Blindness

Centro de Enfermería Diestro (SNF) *n.* Skilled Nursing Facility (SNF)

Centro de Rehabilitación *n.* Rehabilitation Center

Centros Para el Control y la Prevención de Enfermedades (CDC) *n.p.* Centers for Disease Control and Prevention (CDC)

Cerebelar *a.* Cerebellar

Cerebelo *n.* Cerebellum

Cerebro *n.* Brain; *n.* Cerebrum

Cerebro Dividido *n.* Split-Brain

Certificado *a.* Certified

Certificado de Competencia Clínica (CCC) *n.* Certificate of Clinical Competence (CCC)

Cerumen *n.* Cerumen; *n.* Earwax

Cervical *a.* Cervical

Chasquido Consonántico *n.* Click Consonant

Ciencias de la Comunicación *n.p.* Communication Sciences

Cierre *n.* Closure

Cierre Velofaríngeo *n.* Velopharyngeal Closure

Cifosis *n.* Kyphosis

Cilios *n.p.* Cilia

Círculo Arterial Cerebral *n.* Circle of Willis; *n.* Cerebral Arterial Circle

Circunloquio *n.* Circumlocution

Cisura *n.* Fissure

Cisura de Rolando *n.* Fissure of Rolando; *n.* Rolandic Fissure; *n.* Central Sulcus

Cisura de Silvio *n.* Sylvian Fissure; *n.* Lateral Sulcus

Cisura Interhemisférica *n.* Longitudinal Fissure

Claustrum *n.* Claustrum

Clavícula *n*. Clavicle

Clínica Privada *n*. Private Clinic; *n*. Private Practice

Clínica de Otorrinolaringología *n*. Ear, Nose, and Throat Practice (ENT); *n*. Otolaryngology Clinic

Coágulo *n*. Clot

Coalescencia *n*. Coalescence; *n*. Union

Coarticulación *n*. Coarticulation

Cociente *n*. Quotient

Cociente de Abducción *n*. Abduction Quotient

Cóclea *n*. Cochlea

Coda *n*. Coda

Codificación *n*. Codification

Coeficiente de Correlación *n*. Correlation Coefficient

Cognado *n*. Cognate

Cognición *n*. Cognition

Cohesión *n*. Cohesion

Colgajo Retrofaríngeo (PPF) *n.* Posterior Pharyngeal Flap (PPF)

Colículo Inferior *n.* Inferior Colliculus

Collarín Cervical *n.* Cervical Collar; *n.* Neck Brace

Coma *n.* Coma

Comatoso *a.* Comatose

Comisura Anterior *n.* Anterior Commissure

Comisurotomía *n.* Commissurotomy

Comórbido *a.* Comorbid

Comorbilidad *n.* Comorbidity

Competencia *n.* Competence; *n.* Proficiency

Competencia Comunicativa *n.* Communicative Competence

Competencia Cultural *n.* Cultural Competence

Competencia Lingüística *n.* Linguistic Competence

Complejo Olivar Superior (COS) *n.* Superior Olivary Complex (SOC)

Comportamiento *n*. Behavior

Comportamiento Aprendido *n*. Learned Behavior

Comprensión *n*. Comprehension

Comprensión Auditiva *n*. Auditory Comprehension

Comunicación Asistida *n*. Aided Communication

Comunicación Aumentativa y Alternativa (CAA) *n*. Augmentative and Alternative Communication (AAC)

Comunicación Sin Ayuda *n*. Unaided Communication

Comunicación Total (TC) *n*. Total Communication (TC)

Comunicación Verbal *n*. Verbal Communication

Comunidad *n*. Community

Conciencia Corporal *n*. Body Awareness

Concusión *n*. Concussion

Condicionamiento *n*. Conditioning

Condral *a*. Chondral

Conducción Aérea *n*. Air Conduction

Conducción Ósea *n*. Bone Conduction

[189]

Conducta *n.* Conduct; *n.* Behavior

Conducto Auditivo Externo (CAE) *n.* Ear Canal; *n.* External Auditory Meatus (EAM)

Conductos Semicirculares *n.p.* Semicircular Canals; *n.p.* Semicircular Ducts

Confidencialidad *n.* Confidentiality

Congénito *a.* Congenital

Conjugación *n.* Conjugation

Conocimiento *n.* Knowledge

Consciencia Cultural *n.* Cultural Awareness

Consciencia Fonémica *n.* Phonemic Awareness

Consciencia Fonológica *n.* Phonological Awareness

Consejero *n.* Counselor

Consonante *n.* Consonant

Consultorio Privado *n.* Private Practice

Contacto Visual *n.* Eye Contact

Contexto *n.* Context

Contexto Cultural *n.* Cultural Context; *n.* Cultural Environment; *n.* Cultural Background

Contextualización *n.* Contextualization

Continuante *n.* Continuant

Continuidad *n.* Continuity

Continuo de Naturalidad *n.* Continuum of Naturalness

Contracción *n.* Contraction

Contrastar *v.* Contrast

Contrato *n.* Contract

Convulsión *n.* Seizure

Coordinación *n.* Coordination

Coprolalia *n.* Coprolalia

Corchetes *n.* Brackets

Cordectomía *n.* Cordectomy

Corea *n.* Chorea

Coreoatetosis *n.* Choreoathetosis

Corona Radiata *n.* Corona Radiata

Coronal *a.* Coronal

Correlación *n.* Correlation

Corteza *n.* Cortex

Corteza Motora *n.* Motor Cortex

Corteza Prefrontal (PFC) *n.* Prefrontal Cortex (PFC)

Corteza Premotor *n.* Premotor Cortex

Corteza Sensorial *n.* Sensory Cortex

Corteza Somatosensorial *n.* Somatosensory Cortex

Cortical *a.* Cortical

Costilla *n.* Rib

Coxis *n.* Coccyx

Craneal *a.* Cranial

Cráneo *n.* Skull

Craniectomía *n.* Craniectomy

Craniotomía *n.* Craniotomy

Crecimiento Canceroso *n.* Cancerous Growth

Cresta *n.* Crest

Cresta Alveolar *n.* Alveolar Ridge

Crianza *n.* Parenting; *n.* Nurturing

Cricoaritenoide *a.* Cricoarytenoid

Cricofaríngeo *a.* Cricopharyngeal

Cricotiroideo *a.* Cricothyroid

Cromosoma *n.* Chromosome

Crónico *a.* Chronic

Cuerdas Vocales *n.p* Vocal Cords

Cuerdas Vocales Falsas *n.p* False Vocal Cords

Cuerno Anterior (de la Médula Espinal) *n.* Anterior Horn; *n.* Anterior Grey Column

Cuerno Posterior (de la Médula Espinal) *n.* Posterior Horn; *n.* Posterior Grey Column; *n.* Dorsal Horn

Cuerpo Calloso *n.* Corpus Callosum

Cuerpo Celular *n.* Cell Body; *n.* Soma

Cuerpo Estriado *n.* Striatum; *n.* Corpus Striatum; *n.* Striate Nucleus

Cuerpos de Lewy *n.p.* Lewy Bodies

Cuerpos Extranjeros *n.p* Foreign Bodies

Cuidado Continuo *n.* Continuing Care

Cuidado Intensivo *n.* Intensive Care; *n.* Acute Care

Cuidado Intermedio *n.* Intermediate Care

Cuidado Paliativo *n.* Palliative Care

Cuidado Prolongado *n.* Long-Term Care

Cuidado Residencial *n.* Residential Care

D

Daño Neurológico *n.* Neurological Damage

Datos *n.* Data

Decibelio (dB) *n.* Decibel (dB)

Declaración *n.* Declaration; *n.* Utterance

Decúbito *n.* Decubitus

Decúbito Prono *n.* Prone Position

Decúbito Supino *n.* Supine Position

Decussation *n.* Decusación

Defecto del Tubo Neural (DTN) *n.* Neural Tube Defect (NTD)

Defensa *n.* Defense; *n.* Advocacy

Degeneración Lobular Frontotemporal (DLFT) *n.* Frontotemporal Lobar Degeneration (FTLD)

Degeneración Transneuronal *n.* Transneuronal Degeneration

Degeneración Walleriana *n.* Wallerian Degeneration

Degenerativo *a.* Degenerative

Deglución *n.* Swallowing; *n.* Deglutition

Deglución Compensatoria *n.* Compensatory Swallow

Deglución de Bario *n.* Barium Swallow

Deglución Secuencial *n.* Sequential Swallow

Deixis *n.* Deixis

Demencia *n.* Dementia

Demencia con Cuerpos de Lewy *n.* Lewy Body Dementia

Demencia Frontotemporal (DFT) *n.* Frontotemporal Dementia (FTD)

Dendrita *n.* Dendrite

Dental *a.* Dental

Dentición *n.* Dentition

Dentro de Límites Normales (DLN) *a.* Within Normal Limits (WNL)

Departamento de Salud y Servicios Humanos (DHHS) *n.* Department of Health and Human Services (DHHS)

Depresión *n.* Depression

Depresor Lingual *n.* Tongue Depressor

Derivación *n.* Referral

Derivar *v.* Refer

Dermatoma *n.* Dermatome

Derrame *n.* Spillage

Desalineación *n.* Misalignment

Desalineado *a.* Misaligned

Desarrollo *n.* Development

Desarrollo Cognitivo *n.* Cognitive Development

Descendido *a.* Lowered

Descodificación *n.* Decoding

Descriptivismo *n.* Descriptivism; *n.* Descriptive Grammar

Descriptivista *n.* Descriptivist; *a.* Descriptive

Desempeño Lingüístico *n.* Linguistic Performance

Desgarro *n.* Tear

Deshidratar *v*. Dehydrate

Deshidratación *n*. Dehydration

Deslizada *n*. Glide; *a*. Glided

Deslizamiento *n*. Gliding

Desmielinizante *a*. Demyelinating

Desplazamiento *n*. Displacement

Desviación Típica *n*. Standard Deviation

Deterioro *n*. Deterioration; *n*. Impairment

Deterioro Cognitivo Leve (DCL) *n*. Mild Cognitive Impairment (MCI)

Diabetes *n*. Diabetes

Diabético *a*. Diabetic

Diadococinesis *n*. Diadochokinesis

Diafragma *n*. Diaphragm

Diagnosticar *v*. Diagnose

Diagnóstico *n*. Diagnosis

Dialecto *n*. Dialect

Diálisis *n.* Dialysis

Diasquisis *n.* Diaschisis

Didáctico *a.* Didactic; *a.* Teaching; *a.* Educative

Diencéfalo *n.* Diencephalon; *n.* Interbrain

Dientes *n.p.* Teeth

Diéresis *n.* Diaeresis

Dieta *n.* Diet

Dieta Nacional de Disfagia (DND) *n.* National Dysphagia Diet (NDD)

Dietético *a.* Dietary

Dietista *n.* Dietician

Difono *n.* Diphone

Digestión *n.* Digestion

Diglosia *n.* Diglossia

Dígrafo *n.* Digraph

Dilatación *n.* Dilation

Diminutivo *n.* Diminutive

Diptongación *n.* Diphthongization

Diptongo *n.* Diphthong

Disartria *n.* Dysarthria

Disartria Atáxica *n.* Ataxic Dysarthria

Disartria Espástica *n.* Spastic Dysarthria

Disartria Flácida *n.* Flaccid Dysarthria

Disartria Hipercinética *n.* Hyperkinetic Dysarthria

Disartria Hipocinética *n.* Hypokinetic Dysarthria

Disartria Mixta *n.* Mixed Dysarthria

Discapacidad *n.* Disability; *n.* Impairment

Discapacidad Auditiva *n.* Hearing Disability; *n.* Hearing Impairment

Discapacidad del Aprendizaje *n.* Learning Disability

Discapacidad Intelectual *n.* Intellectual Disability (ID)

Discinesia *n.* Dyskinesia

Discinesia Tardía (TD) *n.* Tardive Dyskinesia (TD)

Discriminación *n.* Discrimination

Discriminación por las Discapacidades *n.* Ableism

Disfagia *n.* Dysphagia

Disfagia Esofágica *n.* Esophageal Dysphagia

Disfagia Orofaríngea *n.* Oropharyngeal Dysphagia

Disfluencia *n.* Dysfluency

Disfonía *n.* Dysphonia

Disfonía Espasmódica (SD) *n.* Spasmodic Dysphonia (SD); *n.* Laryngeal Dystonia

Disfonía de Tensión Muscular *n.* Muscle Tension Dysphonia

Disfunción *n.* Dysfunction

Disfuncional *a.* Dysfunctional

Disgrafía *n.* Dysgraphia

Disimilación *n.* Dissimilation

Dislalia *n.* Dyslalia

Dislexia *n.* Dyslexia

Dislocación *n.* Dislocation

Disnea *n.* Dyspnea

[201]

Disortografía *n.* Dysorthography

Disostosis *n.* Dysostosis

Dispepsia *n.* Dyspepsia

Displasia *n.* Dysplasia

Dispositivo *n.* Device

Dispraxia *n.* Dyspraxia

Dispraxia Verbal del Desarrollo (DVD) *n.* Developmental Verbal Dyspraxia (DVD)

Disprosodia *n.* Dysprosody

Distal *a.* Distal

Distinción *n.* Distinction

Distonía *n.* Dystonia

Distonía Laríngea *n.* Laryngeal Dystonia; *n.* Spasmodic Dysphonia (SD)

Distrofia *n.* Dystrophy

Distrofia Muscular *n.* Muscular Dystrophy (MD)

Distrofia Muscular Oculofaríngea *n.* Oculopharyngeal Muscular Dystrophy

Diversidad *n.* Diversity

Divertículo *n.* Diverticulum

Divertículo de Zenker *n.* Zenker's Diverticulum

Divertículos de la Hipofaringe *n.m* Hypopharyngeal Diverticula

Doctor *n.* Doctor; *n.* Physician; *n.* Provider; *n.* Practitioner

Dolor de Garganta *n.* Sore Throat

Dominante *a.* Dominant

Dominio *n.* Proficiency; *n.* Mastery

Dominio Limitado del Inglés (LEP) *n.* Limited English Proficiency (LEP)

Dopamina *n.* Dopamine

Dorsal *a.* Dorsal

Dorso *n.* Dorsum

Duramadre *n.* Dura Mater

E

Ecografía *n.* Ultrasound

Ecolalia *n.* Echolalia

Ectodermo *n.* Ectoderm

Edad *n.* Age

Edad Cronológico *n.* Chronological Age

Edad Escolar *a.* School Age

Edad Gestacional *n.* Gestational Age

Edad Mental *n.* Mental Age

Edad de Desarrollo *n.* Developmental Age

Edadismo *n.* Ageism

Edema *n.* Edema

Edéntulo *a.* Edentulous

Educación Especial *n.* Special Education

Educación por Inmersión *n.* Immersion Education

Eferente *a.* Efferent

Eficacia *n.* Efficacy

Eje *n.* Axis

Electrococleografía (ECoG) *n.* Electrocochleography (ECoG)

Electrodo *n.* Electrode

Electroencefalografía (EEG) *n.* Electroencephalography (EEG)

Elevado *a.* Raised

Elidir *v.* Elide

Elisión *n.* Elision; *n.* Deletion

Embolia *n.* Embolism

Embolia Pulmonar *n.* Pulmonary Embolism

Émbolo *n.* Embolus

Embrión *n.* Embryo

Embrionario *a.* Embryonic

Emisión Nasal *n.* Nasal Emission

Emisión Otoacústica (EOA) *n.* Otoacoustic Emission (OAE)

Empírico *a.* Empirical

Empuje de la Lengua *n.* Tongue Thrust

Encefalitis *n.* Encephalitis

Encefalitis de Rasmussen (ER) *n.* Rasmussen's Encephalitis (RE)

Encefalopatía *n.* Encephalopathy

Encefalopatía Traumática Crónica (ETC) *n.* Chronic Traumatic Encephalopathy (CTE)

Encías *n.p.* Gingiva ; *n.p.* Gums

Endarterectomía Carotídea (EAC) *n.* Carotid Endarterectomy (CEA)

Endodermo *n.* Endoderm

Endógeno *a.* Endogenous

Endolinfa *n.* Endolymph

Endoscópico *a.* Endoscopic

Endoscopio *n.* Endoscope

Enfermedad Autoinmunitaria *n.* Autoimmune Disease

Enfermedad de Alzheimer *n.* Alzheimer's Disease

Enfermedad de Huntington (EH) *n.* Huntington's Disease (HD)

Enfermedad de Ménière *n.* Ménière's Disease (MD)

Enfermedad de Parkinson *n.* Parkinson's Disease

Enfermedad de Pica *n.* Pica

Enfermedad de Transmisión Sexual (ETS) *n.* Sexually Transmitted Disease (STD); *n.* Sexually Transmitted Infection (STI)

Enfermedad Pulmonar Obstructiva Crónica (EPOC) *n.* Chronic Obstructive Pulmonary Disease (COPD)

Enfermedad por Reflujo Gastroesofágico (ERGE) *n.* Gastroesophageal Reflux Disease (GERD)

Enfoque *n.* Focus; *n.* Approach

Enseñanza Ambiental Mejorada (EMT) *n.* Enhanced Milieu Teaching (EMT)

Enseñanza Incidental *n.* Incidental Teaching

Ensordecimiento *n.* Devoicing

Entonación *n.* Intonation

Entorno Educativo *n.* Educational Environment

Entrenamiento *n.* Training; *n.* Coaching

Entrevista *n.* Interview

Enunciado *n.* Utterance

Enunciado Performativo *n.* Performative Utterance

Envejecimiento *n.* Aging

Enzima *n.* Enzyme

Epéndimocitos *n.p.* Epyndemal Cells

Epéntesis *n.* Epenthesis

Epidural *a.* Epidural

Epiglotis *n.* Epiglottis

Epilepsia *n.* Epilepsy

Equipo *n.* Team

Equipo de la Alimentación *n.* Feeding Team

Errores de Articulación *n.* Misarticulation; *n.* Articulation Errors

Escala de Coma de Glasgow *n.* Glasgow Coma Scale (GCS)

Escala de Penetración-Aspiración (PAS) *n.* Penetration-Aspiration Scale (PAS)

Escaneo *n.* Scan; *n.* Scanning

Escápula *n.* Scapula

Escintigrafía *n.* Scintigraphy

Esclerosis Lateral Amiotrófica (ELA) *n.* Amyotrophic Lateral Sclerosis (ALS); *n.* Lou Gehrig's Disease

Esclerosis Múltiple *n.* Multiple Sclerosis

Escoliosis *n.* Scoliosis

Escuela Primaria *n.* Primary School; *n.* Elementary School

Escuela Privada *n.* Private School

Escuela Pública *n.* Public School

Escuela Secundaria *n.* High School; *n.* Middle School; *n.* Secondary School

Esdrújula *a.* Proparoxytone

Esfínter *n.* Sphincter

Esfínter Esofágico Inferior (EEI) *n.* Lower Esophageal Sphincter (LES)

Esfínter Esofágico Superior (EES) *n.* Upper Esophageal Sphincter (UES); *n.* Segmento Faringoesofágico

Esfuerzo Vocal *n.* Vocal Strain

Esofagectomía *n.* Esophagectomy

Esofagitis *n.* Esophagitis

Esofagitis Eosinofílica *n.* Eosinophilic Esophagitis

Esofagitis por Reflujo *n.* Reflux Esophagitis

Esófago *n.* Esophagus

Esofagografía con Bario *n.* Barium Swallow; *n.* Modified Barium Swallow Study (MBSS)

Espasmo *n.* Spasm

Espasmo Esofágico Difuso *n.* Diffuse Esophageal Spasm

Espasticidad *n.* Spasticity

Espástico *a.* Spastic

Especialista *n.* Specialist

Espectro *n.* Spectrum

Espectrograma *n.* Spectrogram

Espina Bífida *n.* Spina Bifida

Espiración de Aire *n.* Expiration of Air

Espirante *n.* Spirant; *a.* Spirant

Espirantización *n.* Spirantization

Espondeo *n.* Spondee

Espontáneo *a.* Spontaneous

Estadística *n.* Statistic

Estadísticamente Significativo *a.* Statistically Significant

Estado *n.* Status; *n.* State

Estandarizado *a.* Standardized

Estenosis *n.* Stenosis; *n.* Stricture

Estenosis Esofágica *n.* Esophageal Stricture

Estereocilia *n.* Stereocilia

Esternón *n.* Sternum

Estetoscopio *n.* Stethoscope

Estigma *n.* Stigma

Estigmatizado *a.* Stigmatized

Estilo de Aprendizaje *n.* Learning Style

Estimulación Cerebral Profunda (DBS) *n.* Deep Brain Stimulation (DBS)

Estímulo *n.* Stimulus

Estoma *n.* Stoma

Estrategia *n.* Strategy

Estrategias Compensatorias *n.p.* Compensatory Strategies

Estreñimiento *n.* Constipation

Estribo *n.* Stapes

Estridente *n.* Strident

Estridor *n.* Stridor

Estroboscopia *n.* Stroboscopy

Estroboscopia Laríngea *n*. Laryngeal Stroboscopy

Estudio de Caso *n*. Case Study

Estudio de Cohorte *n*. Cohort Study

Estudio Longitudinal *n*. Longitudinal Study

Etapa *n*. Stage; *n*. Phase

Etapa Operacional Concreta *n*. Concrete Operational Stage

Etapa Operacional Formal *n*. Formal Operational Stage

Etapa Preoperativa *n*. Preoperational Stage

Etapa Sensomotora *n*. Sensorimotor Stage

Etapas de Deglución *n.p.* Stages of Swallowing; *n.p.* Phases of Swallowing

Ética *n*. Ethics

Etimología *n*. Etymology

Etiología *n*. Etiology

Etnográfico *a*. Ethnographic

Etnolingüístico *a*. Ethnolinguistic

Eupnea *n.* Eupnea

Evaluación *n.* Evaluation; *n.* Assessment

Evaluación Dinámica (ED) *n.* Dynamic Assessment

Evaluación Endoscópica de la Deglución por Fibra Óptica (FEES) *n.* Fiberoptic Endoscopic Evaluation of Swallowing (FEES)

Evaluación Endoscópica Flexible de la Deglución con Pruebas Sensoriales (FEESST) *n.* Flexible Endoscopic Evaluation of Swallowing with Sensory Testing (FEESST)

Evaluación Formativa *n.* Formative Assessment

Evaluación Observacional *n.* Observational Assessment

Evaluación Predictiva *n.* Predictive Assessment

Evaluación Sumativa *n.* Summative Assessment

Evocación de Palabras *n.* Word Finding; *n.* Word Retrieval

Exacerbación *n.* Exacerbation

Exactitud *n.* Accuracy

Examen *n.* Examination; *n.* Test; *n.* Screening

Examen al Lado del Paciente *n.* Bedside Examination

Examen Periférico Oral *n.* Oral Peripheral Examination

Exógeno *a.* Exogenous

Expansión *n.* Expansion

Expectorar *v.* Expectorate

Expresión *n.* Expression; *n.* Utterance

Extender *v.* Extend

Extensión *n.* Extension

Externo *a.* External

Extrahospitalario *a.* Outpatient

Extrapiramidal *a.* Extrapyramidal

F

Facilitar *v.* Facilitate

Factor Desencadenante *n.* Precipitating Factor; *n.* Triggering Factor

Factor de Riesgo *n.* Risk Factor

Fallecer *v.* Pass Away; *v.* Decease; *v.* Perish

Faringe *n.* Pharynx

Faringealización *n.* Pharyngealization

Faríngeo *a.* Pharyngeal

Faringoplastia *n.* Pharyngoplasty

Farmacéutico *a.* Pharmaceutical

Fármacos *n.* Drugs; *n.* Pharmaceuticals

Fasciculación *n.* Fasciculation

Fascículo *n.* Fasciculus

Fascículo Arqueado *n.* Arcuate Fasciculus

Fase Esofágica *n.* Esophageal Phase

Fase Faríngea *n*. Pharyngeal Phase

Fase Oral *n*. Oral Phase

Fase Oral Preparatoria *n*. Oral Preparatory Phase

Fatiga *n*. Fatigue

Fatiga Vocal *n*. Vocal Fatigue

Fetal *a*. Fetal

Feto *n*. Fetus

Fibroscopio *n*. Fiberscope

Fibrosis Quística *n*. Cystic Fibrosis

Ficha del Paciente *n*. Patient Chart; *n*. Patient Medical Record

Firmeza *n*. Steadiness

Fisiología *n*. Physiology

Fisiológico *a*. Physiological

Fisiopatología *n*. Pathophysiology

Fisioterapeuta *n*. Physical Therapist

Fisioterapia *n*. Physical Therapy

Fístula *n.* Fistula

Fístula Traqueoesofágica *n.* Tracheoesophageal Fistula

Flacidez *n.* Flaccidity

Flexión *n.* Flexion; *n.* Inflection

Flexionar *v.* Flex

Fluidez *n.* Fluency

Fluidez del Habla *n.* Fluency of Speech

Fluido *a.* Fluent

Flujo de Aire *n.* Airflow

Fluoroscopia *n.* Fluoroscopy

Fobia *n.* Phobia

Fonación *n.* Phonation

Fonema *n.* Phoneme

Fonestema *n.* Phonestheme

Fonética Articulatoria *n.* Articulatory Phonetics

Fonético *a.* Phonetic

Fonoaudiología *n.* Speech-Language Pathology; *n.* Phonoaudiology

Fonoaudiólogo *n.* Speech-Language Pathologist; *n.* Phonoaudiologist

Fonología *n.* Phonology

Fonotáctica *n.* Phonotactics

Foramen *n.* Foramen

Foramen Magno *n.* Foramen Magnum

Formación Reticular (FR) *n.* Reticular Formation (RF)

Formante *n.* Formant

Fortición *n.* Fortition

Frase *n.* Sentence; *n.* Phrase

Frecuencia *n.* Frequency

Frecuencia de Aparición *n.* Frequency of Occurrence

Frecuencia Fundamental *n.* Fundamental Frequency

Frenillo *n.* Frenulum; *n.* Frenum

Fricativa *n.* Fricative; *a.* Fricative

[219]

Fuente *n.* Source

Funcional *a.* Functional

Función Ejecutiva *n.* Executive Function

G

Galleta *n.* Cracker; *n.* Cookie

Gama *n.* Spectrum; *n.* Range

Gammagrafía *n.* Scintigraphy

Ganglio *n.* Node; *n.* Ganglion

Ganglios Basales *n.p.* Basal Ganglia

Ganglios Espinales *n.p.* Spinal Ganglia; *n.p.* Dorsal Root Ganglia

Gástrico *a.* Gastric

Gastroesofágico *a.* Gastroesophageal

Gastrostomía *n.* Gastrostomy

Gastrostomía Endoscópica Percutánea (GEP) *n.* Percutaneous Endoscopic Gastrostomy (PEG)

Geminación *n.* Gemination

Gen *n.* Gene

Generalizar *v.* Generalize

Genérico *a.* Generic

Genético *a*. Genetic

Geriátrico *n*. Nursing Home

Gestación *n*. Gestation

Gestalt *n*. Gestalt

Gesto *n*. Gesture

Gesto Antagonista *n*. Sensory Trick; *n*. Geste Antagoniste

Giro *n*. Gyrus

Giro Angular *n*. Angular Gyrus

Giro Cingulado *n*. Cingulate Gyrus

Giro de Heschl *n*. Heschl's Gyrus; *n*. Transverse Temporal Gyrus

Giro Fusiforme *n*. Fusiform Gyrus

Giro Parahipocampal *n*. Parahippocampal Gyrus

Giro Poscentral *n*. Post-Central Gyrus

Giro Precentral *n*. Precentral Gyrus

Giro Supramarginal *n*. Supramarginal Gyrus

Glándula *n*. Gland

Glándula Pituitaria *n.* Pituitary Gland

Glándula Salival *n.* Salivary Gland

Glándula Tiroides *n.* Thyroid Gland

Glioma *n.* Glioma

Globo *n.* Globus

Globo Pálido *n.* Globus Pallidus

Glosectomía *n.* Glossectomy

Glosolalia *n.* Glossolalia

Glotal *a.* Glottal

Glotis *n.* Glottis

Grado *n.* Degree

Grafema *n.* Grapheme

Gramática *n.* Grammar

Gramática Generativa *n.* Generative Grammar

Gramática Generativa Transformacional *n.* Transformational Grammar

Grave *a.* Severe; *a.* Acute

Grupo Consonántico *n.* Consonant Cluster; *n.* Consonant Blend

Grupo de Apoyo *n.* Support Group

Grupo de Autoayuda *n.* Self-Help Group

Guardería *n.* Day Care; *n.* Nursery; *n.* Child Care Center; *n.* Kindergarten

H

Habilidades Sociales *n.p.* Social Skills

Habilitación *n.* Habilitation

Habla *n.* Speech

Habla Digitalizada *n.* Digitized Speech

Habla Entrecortada *n.* Bumpy Speech; *n.* Choppy Speech

Habla Escandida *n.* Scanning Speech

Habla Irregular *n.* Irregular Speech; *n.* Bumpy Speech

Habla Lenta *n.* Slow Speech

Habla Modificada *n.* Modified Speech; *n.* Altered Speech

Habla Telegráfica *n.* Telegraphic Speech

Hablante de Herencia *n.* Heritage Speaker

Hablante Tardío *n.* Late Talker

Hacer Señas *v.* Sign; *n.* Signing

Hélice *n.* Helix

Helicotrema *n.* Helicotrema

Hemianopsia *n.* Hemianopsia

Hemibalismo *n.* Hemiballism

Hemicránea *n.* Hemicrania; *n.* Migraine

Hemiparesia *n.* Hemiparesis

Hemiplejia *n.* Hemiplegia

Hemisferio (Izquierdo o Derecho) *n.* Hemisphere (Left or Right)

Hemorragia *n.* Hemorrhage

Hendidura *n.* Cleft

Hercio (Hz) *n.* Hertz (Hz)

Heredado *a.* Inherited

Heredar *v.* Inherit

Hereditario *a.* Hereditary

Herida por Arma de Fuego *n.* Gunshot Wound (GSW)

Hernia *n.* Hernia

Heterogéneo *a.* Heterogeneous

Hiato *n.* Hiatus

Hidrocefalia *n.* Hydrocephalus

Hidrocefalia Normotensiva (HNT) *n.* Normal Pressure Hydrocephalus (NPH)

Hidrops Endolinfático *n.* Endolymphatic Hydrops

Hinchado *a.* Swollen

Hinchazón *n.* Swelling

Hipercinesia *n.* Hyperkinesia

Hipercinético *a.* Hyperkinetic

Hipercorrección *n.* Hypercorrection

Hiperextranjerismo *n.* Hyperforeignism

Hiperflexión *n.* Hyperflexion

Hipernasal *a.* Hypernasal

Hiperperfusión *n.* Hyperperfusion

Hiperreflexia *n.* Hyperreflexia

Hipertensión (HTN) *n.* Hypertension (HTN); *n.* High Blood Pressure (HBP)

Hipertiroidismo *n.* Hyperthyroidism

Hipertonía *n.* Hypertonia

Hipertónico *n.* Hypertonic

Hipo *n.* Hiccup

Hipocampo *n.* Hippocampus

Hipocinesia *n.* Hypokinesia

Hipofaringe *n.* Hypopharynx

Hiponasal *a.* Hyponasal

Hipoperfusión *n.* Hypoperfusion

Hipotálamo *n.* Hypothalamus

Hipótesis *n.* Hypothesis

Hipótesis Nula *n.* Null Hypothesis

Hipotiroidismo *n.* Hypothyroidism

Hipotónico *a.* Hypotonic

Hipoxia *n.* Hypoxia

Historia Médica *n.* Medical History; *n.* Medical Chart; *n.* Case History

Holístico *a.* Holistic

Holoprosencefalia (HPE) *n.* Holoprosencephaly (HPE)

Homeostasis *n.* Homeostasis

Homogéneo *a.* Homogenous

Homúnculo *n.* Homunculus

Hospicio *n.* Hospice

Hospitalización *n.* Hospitalization

Huesecillo *n.* Ossicle

Hueso Hioides *n.* Hyoid Bone

I

Ictus *n.* Stroke; *n.* Cerebrovascular Accident (CVA)

Ictus Embólico *n.* Embolic Stroke

Ictus Hemorrágico *n.* Hemorrhagic Stroke

Ictus Isquémico *n.* Ischemic Stroke; *n.* Occlusive Stroke

Ictus Trombótico *n.* Thrombotic Stroke

Idiolecto *n.* Idiolect

Idioma *n.* Language

Idiomático *a.* Idiomatic

Idiosincrático *a.* Idiosyncratic

Idiotismo *n.* Idiom

Ilion *n.* Ilium

Ilocutivo *a.* Illocutionary

Imagen por Resonancia Magnética (IRM) *n.* Magnetic Resonance Imaging (MRI)

Imagen por Resonancia Magnética Funcional (IRMf) *n.* Functional Magnetic Resonance Imaging (fMRI)

Imágenes *n.p.* Images; *n.* Imaging

Imitación *n.* Imitation

Impedancia *n.* Impedance

Impedanciometría *n.* Impedanciometry

Implante Auditivo Osteointegrado (AOI) *n.* Bone-Anchored Hearing Aid (BAHA); *n.* Bone-Anchored Hearing Implant (BAHI)

Implante Auditivo de Tronco Cerebral (IATC) *n.* Auditory Brainstem Implant (ABI)

Implante Coclear *n.* Cochlear Implant

Inadaptado *a.* Maladaptive

Incidencia *n.* Incidence

Incisivos *n.p.* Incisors

Inclusión *n.* Inclusion

Incompetencia *n.* Incompetence

Incontinencia Afectiva *n.* Pseudobulbar Affect (PBA); *n.* Emotional Incontinence; *n.* Emotional Lability

Incorporación *n.* Incorporation; *n.* Mainstreaming; *n.* Inclusion

Inducción *n.* Induction

Inervación *n.* Innervation

Infante *n.* Infant

Infantil *a.* Infantile

Infarto *n.* Infarct; *n.* Heart Attack

Infarto Agudo de Miocardio (IAM) *n.* Acute Myocardial Infarction (AMI); *n.* Heart Attack

Infección *n.* Infection

Inferior *a.* Lower; *a.* Inferior

Inflamación *n.* Inflammation; *n.* Swelling

Ingesta Dietética *n.* Dietary Intake

Ingestión *n.* Ingestion

Inglés Afroestadounidense Vernáculo (IAV) *n.* African-American Vernacular English (AAVE)

Inglés Como Lengua Extranjera (EFL) *n.* English as a Foreign Language (EFL)

Inglés como Segunda Lengua (ESL) *n.* English as a Second Language (ESL)

Inhalador *n.* Inhaler

Inhalar *v.* Inhale

Inicio *n.* Onset; *n.* Start

Inicio Suave *n.* Easy Onset

Injerto *n.* Graft

Inmitancia *n.* Immittance

Inmunidad *n.* Immunity

Inmunización *n.* Immunization

Innato *a.* Innate

Insonoro *a.* Voiceless

Inspirar Aire *v.* Inspire Air

Insuficiencia Velofaríngea *n.* Velopharyngeal Insufficiency (VPI); *n.* Velopharyngeal Dysfunction (VPD)

Insuficiencia Vertebrobasilar (IVB) *n.* Vertebrobasilar Insufficiency (VBI)

Ínsula *n.* Insula

Integración *n.* Integration; *n.* Inclusion

Inteligibilidad *n.* Intelligibility

Intensidad *n.* Intensity

Intensidad Vocal *n.* Vocal Intensity

Intento Comunicativo *n.* Communicative Intent

Interaccionista *a.* Interactionist

Intercambiabilidad *n.* Interchangeability

Interdental *a.* Interdental

Interferencia *n.* Interference

Interfijo *n.* Interfix

Interjección *n.* Interjection

Interlengua *n.* Interlanguage

Interlocutor *n.* Interlocutor

Intermedio *a.* Intermediate

Intermitente *a.* Intermittent

Interno *a.* Internal

Intérprete *n.* Interpreter

Intervalo Aéreo-Óseo *n.* Air-Bone Gap

Intervalo de Confianza *n.* Confidence Interval

Intervención *n.* Intervention

Intervención Rápida *n.* Early Intervention

Intrahospitalario *a.* Inpatient

Invasivo *a.* Invasive

Inventario *n.* Inventory

Investigación *n.* Research

Inyección *n.* Injection

IRM de Difusión *n.* Diffusion MRI

Irreversible *a.* Irreversible

Isquemia *n.* Ischemia

Isquion *n.* Ischium

Istmo de las Fauces *n.* Fauces

J

Jaqueca *n.* Migraine; *n.* Headache

Jardín de Infantes *n.* Kindergarten; *n.* Nursery

Jerga *n.* Jargon

Jitter *n.* Jitter; *n.* Fluctuación

Juego Cooperativo *n.* Cooperative Play

Juego Simbólico *n.* Symbolic Play

Juventud *n.* Youth

K

Kindergarten *n.* Kindergarten

Kinesiología *n.* Kinesiology

Kinesiólogo *n.* Kinesiologist

L

La Palabra Complementada (LPC) *n.* Cued Speech

Laberintitis *n.* Labyrinthitis

Laberinto Óseo *n.* Bony Labyrinth; *n.* Osseous Labyrinth

Labial *a.* Labial

Labialización *n.* Labialization

Labilidad Emocional *n.* Emotional Lability

Labio Leporino *n.* Cleft Lip

Labiodental *a.* Labiodental

Labios *n.* Lips; *n.* Labia

Labiovelar *a.* Labiovelar

Lactación *n.* Lactation; *n.* Suckling; *n.* Nursing; *n.* Breastfeeding

Lámina *n.* Lamina

Lámina Espiral Ósea *n.* Osseous Spiral Lamina

Laminar *a.* Laminal

Laringe *n.* Larynx; *n.* Voice Box

Laringectomía *n.* Laryngectomy

Laríngeo *a.* Laryngeal

Laringitis *n.* Laryngitis

Laringocele *n.* Laryngocele

Laringoespasmo *n.* Laryngospasm

Laringógrafo (EGG) *n.* Electroglottography (EGG)

Laringólogo *n.* Laryngologist

Laringomalacia *n.* Laryngomalacia

Laringoplastia *n.* Laryngoplasty

Laringoscopía *n.* Laryngoscopy

Laringoscopio *n.* Laryngoscope

Láser *n.* Laser

Lateral *n.* Lateral; *a.* Lateral

Lateralidad *n.* Laterality

Lectura Labial *n.* Lip Reading

Lema *n.* Lemma

Lemnisco *n.* Lemniscus

Lengua *n.* Tongue; *n.* Language

Lengua Criolla *n.* Creole Language

Lengua de Signos *n.* Sign Language

Lengua de Signos Americana (ASL) *n.* American Sign Language (ASL)

Lenguaje *n.* Language

Lenguaje Expresivo *n.* Expressive Language

Lenguaje Figurativo *n.* Figurative Language

Lenguaje Formuláico *n.* Formulaic Language

Lenguaje Funcional *n.* Functional Language

Lenguaje Precipitado *n.* Hurried Language; *n.* Cluttered Language; *n.* Cluttering

Lenguaje Proposicional/ No Proposicional *n.* Propositional/ Non-Propositional Language

Lenguaje Receptivo *n.* Receptive Language

Lenguaje de Bebé *n.* Baby Talk; *n.* Motherese

Lenición *n.* Lenition

Lesión *n.* Lesion; *n.* Injury; *n.* Damage

Lesión Cerebral Adquirida (LCA) *n.* Acquired Brain Injury (ABI)

Lesión Cerebral Traumática (LCT) *n.* Traumatic Brain Injury (TBI)

Lesión Craneal Abierta *n.* Open Head Injury (OHI)

Lesión Craneal Cerrada *n.* Closed Head Injury (CHI)

Lesión de la Médula Espinal (LME) *n.* Spinal Cord Injury (SCI)

Leucoplasia *n.* Leukoplakia

Leve *a.* Mild

Léxico *a.* Lexical; *n.* Lexicon

Ley Para la Educación de Individuos con Discapacidades (IDEA) *n.* Individuals with Disabilities Education Act (IDEA)

Ley Sobre Estadounidenses con Discapacidades (ADA) *n.* Americans with Disabilities Act (ADA)

Liberación Miofascial *n.* Myofascial Release

Ligamento *n.* Ligament

Limitación *n.* Limitation

Linfa *n.* Lymph

Lingua Franca *n.* Lingua Franca

Lingual *a.* Lingual

Lingüística *n.* Linguistics

Lingüística Aplicada *n.* Applied Linguistics

Linguolabial *a.* Linguolabial

Líquido *n.* Liquid; *n.* Fluid; *a.* Liquid

Líquido Cerebroespinal (LCE) *n.* Cerebrospinal Fluid (CSF)

Líquido Fino *n.* Thin Liquid; *n.* Thin Fluid

Lisencefalia *n.* Lissencephaly

Llana *a.* Paroxytone

Lóbulo *n.* Lobe

Lóbulo Frontal *n.* Frontal Lobe

Lóbulo Parietal *n.* Parietal Lobe

Lóbulo Temporal *n.* Temporal Lobe

Localización *n.* Localization

Logoaudiometría *n.* Speech Audiometry

Logopeda *n.* Speech Therapist; *n.* Speech Pathologist

Logopedia *n.* Speech Therapy; *n.* Logopedics; *n.* Speech-Language Pathology

Logorrea *n.* Logorrhea

Longitud de Onda *n.* Wavelength

Longitudinal *a.* Longitudinal

Lordosis *n.* Lordosis

Lumen *n.* Lumen

Lumen Esofágico *n.* Esophageal Lumen

M

Macrocefalia *n.* Macrocephaly

Macroglosia *n.* Macroglossia

Mal Articulado *a.* Slurred; *a.* Poorly Articulated

Mala Articulación *n.* Slurring; *n.* Poor Articulation

Malformación *n.* Malformation

Malformación Arteriovenosa (MAV) *n.* Arteriovenous Malformation (AVM)

Malformación de Chiari *n.* Chiari Malformation

Maligno *a.* Malignant

Maloclusión *n.* Malocclusion

Mandíbula *n.* Jaw; *n.* Mandible

Mandibular *a.* Mandibular

Mandibulofacial *a.* Mandibulofacial

Manometría Esofágica *n.* Esophageal Manometry

Manómetro *n.* Manometer

Manzana de Adán *n.* Adam's Apple

Mapeo *n.* Mapping

Marcación *n.* Labelling; *n.* Marking

Marcado *a.* Marked

Marcador de Caso *n.* Case Marker

Martillo *n.* Malleus

Masticación *n.* Mastication; *n.* Chewing

Masticado *a.* Masticated; *a.* Chewed

Mastoideo *a.* Mastoid

Maternés *n.* Motherese

Maxilar *n.* Maxilla

Meaning *n.* Significado

Mecanismo del Habla *n.* Speech Mechanism

Mecanismo Velofaríngeo (MV) *n.* Velopharyngeal Port (VPP); Velopharyngeal Sphincter

Medial *a.* Medial; *a.* Midsagittal

Mediastino *n.* Mediastinum

Medicamentos *n.p.* Medications; *n.p.* Drugs

Mediosagital *a.* Midsagittal

Médula Espinal *n.* Spinal Cord

Mejoría *n.* Improvement

Membrana *n.* Membrane

Membrana Basilar *n.* Basilar Membrane

Membrana Mucosa *n.* Mucous Membrane

Membrana Timpánica *n.* Tympanic Membrane; *n.* Eardrum

Membranoso *a.* Membranous

Memoria *n.* Memory

Memoria a Corto Plazo (MCP) *n.* Short-Term Memory

Memoria a Largo Plazo (MLP) *n.* Long-Term Memory (LTM)

Memoria de Trabajo *n.* Working Memory

Memoria Episódica *n.* Episodic Memory

Memoria Explícita *n.* Explicit Memory; *n.* Declarative Memory

Memoria Implícita *n.* Implicit Memory

Memoria Procedimental *n.* Procedural Memory

Memoria Semántica *n.* Semantic Memory

Meninge *n.* Meninge

Meningitis *n.* Meningitis

Mentor *n.* Mentor

Mesencéfalo *n.* Mesencephalon; *n.* Midbrain

Mesodermo *n.* Mesoderm

Mesotelial *a.* Mesothelial

Mesotelioma *n.* Mesothelioma

Meta *n.* Goal; *n.* Target

Metabolismo *n.* Metabolism

Metacognición *n.* Metacognition

Metáfora *n.* Metaphor

Metalingüístico *a.* Metalinguistic

Metástasis *n.* Metastasis

Metátesis *n.* Metathesis

Metencéfalo *n.* Metencephalon

Método Silábico *n.* Phonics

Miastenia Grave (MG) *n.* Myasthenia Gravis (MG)

Microcefalia *n.* Microcephaly

Microglía *n.p.* Microglia

Micrognacia *n.* Micrognathia

Microscópico *a.* Microscopic

Microscopio *n.* Microscope

Microsomía *n.* Microsomia

Microtia *n.* Microtia

Miel *n.* Honey

Mielina *n.* Myelin

Mielencéfalo *n.* Myelencephalon

Migraña *n.* Migraine

Mínimamente Invasivo *a*. Minimally Invasive

Minoría *n*. Minority

Mioclono *n*. Myoclonus

Miofuncional *a*. Myofunctional

Miotoma *n*. Myotome

Mirada *n*. Gaze; *n*. Eye Gaze

Miringotomía *n*. Myringotomy

Mitigar *v*. Mitigate

Modales *n*. Bedside Manner

Modalidad *n*. Modality

Modelación *n*. Modeling

Modelación de la Fluidez *n*. Fluency Shaping

Modelo Fuente-Filtro de la Voz *n*. Source-Filter Model

Modelo Mand *n*. Mand-Model Approach

Moderado *a*. Moderate

Modificación *n*. Shaping; *n*. Modification

Modiolo n. Modiolus

Modo de Articulación n. Manner of Articulation

Molares n. Molars

Monolingüe a. Monolingual

Monólogo n. Monologue

Monosilábico a. Monosyllabic

Morbilidad n. Morbidity

Mordida n. Bite

Mordida Abierta n. Open Bite

Mordida Fásica n. Phasic Bite

Morfema n. Morpheme

Morfema Libre n. Free Morpheme

Morfema Ligado n. Bound Morpheme

Morfología n. Morphology

Motoneurona (Superior/Inferior) n. (Upper/Lower) Motor Neuron

Motora Oral a. Oral Motor

Motricidad *n.p.* Motor Skills

Motricidad Fina *n.p.* Fine Motor Skills

Motricidad Gruesa *n.p.* Gross Motor Skills

Movimiento *n.* Movement

Mucosa *n.* Mucosa

Mudo *a.* Mute; *a.* Silent

Muestra *n.* Sample

Muestra Aleatoria *n.* Random Sample

Muestra de Lenguaje *n.* Language Sample

Muestreo *n.* Sampling

Muletilla *n.* Filler

Multicultural *a.* Multicultural

Multilingüe *a.* Multilingual

Multimodalidad *n.* Multimodality

Músculo *n.* Muscle

Músculo Buceador *n.* Buccinator Muscle

Músculo Cutáneo *n.* Platysma Muscle

Músculo Digástrico *n.* Digastric Muscle

Músculo Esquelético *n.* Skeletal Muscle

Músculo Estapedio *n.* Stapedius

Músculo Estriado *n.* Striated Muscle

Músculo Liso *n.* Smooth Muscle

Músculo Masetero *n.* Masseter Muscle

Músculo Orbicular de la Boca *n.* Orbicularis Oris Muscle

Músculo Platisma *n.* Platysma Muscle

Músculo Pterigoideo *n.* Pterygoid Muscle

Músculo Tensor del Tímpano *n.* Tensor Tympani

Músculos Infrahioideos *n.p* Infrahyoid Muscles

Músculos Suprahioideos *n.p* Suprahyoid Muscles

Mutación *n.* Mutation

Mutismo *n.* Mutism

Mutismo Selectivo (SM) *n.* Selective Mutism (SM)

N

Nada por Vía Oral/Nil per os (NPO) *a.* Nothing by Mouth/Nil per os (NPO)

Narración *n.* Narration

Nasal *a.* Nasal

Nasalidad *n.* Nasality

Nasalización *n.* Nasalization

Nasofaringe *n.* Nasopharynx

Nasogástrico (NG) *a.* Nasogastric (NG)

Nasometría *n.* Nasometry

Nativista *a.* Nativist

Nativización *n.* Nativization

Nativo *a.* Native

Naturalista *a.* Naturalist

Necrosis *n.* Necrosis

Néctar *n.* Nectar

Negación *n.* Negation; *n.* Denial

Negligencia *n.* Negligence; *n.* Neglect

Neonatal *a.* Neonatal

Neoplasia *n.* Neoplasm

Nervio *n.* Nerve

Nervio Abducens *n.* Abducens Nerve

Nervio Accesorio *n.* Accessory Nerve

Nervio Coclear *n.* Cochlear Nerve; *n.* Auditory Nerve; *n.* Acoustic Nerve

Nervio Craneal *n.* Cranial Nerve

Nervio Espinal Accesorio *n.* Accessory Nerve

Nervio Estatoacústico *n.* Vestibulocochlear Nerve

Nervio Facial *n.* Facial Nerve

Nervio Faríngeo *n.* Pharyngeal Nerve

Nervio Frénico *n.* Phrenic Nerve

Nervio Glosofaríngeo *n.* Glossopharyngeal Nerve

Nervio Hipogloso *n.* Hypoglossal Nerve

Nervio Laríngeo Recurrente (NLR) *n*. Recurrent Laryngeal Nerve (RLN)

Nervio Laríngeo Superior (NLS) *n*. Superior Laryngeal Nerve (SLN)

Nervio Motor Ocular Común (MOC) *n*. Oculomotor Nerve

Nervio Motor Ocular Externo (MOT) *n*. Abducens Nerve

Nervio Neumogástrico *n*. Vagus Nerve; *n*. Pneumogastric Nerve

Nervio Ocular *n*. Optic Nerve

Nervio Oculomotor *n*. Oculomotor Nerve

Nervio Olfativo *n*. Olfactory Nerve

Nervio Óptico *n*. Optic Nerve

Nervio Patético *n*. Trochlear Nerve

Nervio Trigémino *n*. Trigeminal Nerve

Nervio Troclear *n*. Trochlear Nerve

Nervio Vago *n*. Vagus Nerve

Nervio Vestibular *n*. Vestibular Nerve

Nervio Vestibulococlear *n.* Vestibulocochlear Nerve

Neumonía *n.* Pneumonia

Neumonía por Aspiración *n.* Aspiration Pneumonia

Neumonitis *n.* Pneumonitis

Neumonitis por Aspiración *n.* Aspiration Pneumonitis

Neumotórax *n.* Pneumothorax

Neurinoma del Acústico *n.* Acoustic Neuroma; *n.* Vestibular Schwannoma

Neurodegenerativo *a.* Neurodegenerative

Neurodiversidad *n.* Neurodiversity

Neurogénesis *n.* Neurogenesis

Neurolingüística *n.* Neurolinguistics

Neurólogo *n.* Neurologist

Neurona *n.* Neuron

Neurona Motora *n.* Motor Neuron

Neurona Motora Inferior (NMI) *n.* Lower Motor Neuron (LMN)

Neurona Motora Superior (NMS) *n.* Upper Motor Neuron (UMN)

Neuroplasticidad *n.* Neuroplasticity

Neurotípico *a.* Neurotypical

Neurotransmisor *n.* Neurotransmitter

Neurulación *n.* Neurulation

Neutral *a.* Neutral

Neutral en Cuanto al Género *a.* Gender-Neutral

Neutralización *n.* Neutralization

Neutralizar *v.* Neutralize

Nistagmo *n.* Nystagmus

Nivelación *n.* Levelling

No Marcado *a.* Unmarked

No Redondeada *a.* Unrounded

No Verbal *a.* Nonverbal

Nodo de Ranvier *n.* Node of Ranvier

Nódulo *n.* Nodule

Nombramiento *n.* Naming

Normativismo *n.* Prescriptivism; *n.* Normativism; *n.* Prescriptive Grammar

Normativo *a.* Normative

Notocorda *n.* Notochord

Núcleo *n.* Nucleus; *n.* Body

Núcleo Caudado *n.* Caudate Nucleus

Núcleo Coclear *n.* Cochlear Nucleus

Núcleo Geniculado Lateral *n.* Lateral Geniculate Nucleus; *n.* Lateral Geniculate Body

Núcleo Geniculado Medial *n.* Medial Geniculate Nucleus; *n.* Medial Geniculate Body

Nuez de Adán *n.* Adam's Apple

Nutrición *n.* Nutrition

Nutrición Enteral *n.* Enteral Nutrition

Nutrición Parenteral *n.* Parenteral Nutrition

Nutrición Parenteral Total (NPT) *n.* Total Parenteral Nutrition (TPN)

O

Observación *n.* Observation; *n.* Shadowing

Obstrucción *n.* Obstruction; *n.* Blocking

Obstruir *v.* Obstruct

Obstruyente *n.* Obstruent; *a.* Obstruent

Obturador *n.* Obturator

Oclusión *n.* Occlusion; *n.* Bite

Oclusión Dental *n.* Dental Occlusion

Oclusiva *n.* Occlusive; *a.* Occlusive; *n.* Plosive; *n.* Stop

Oclusivización *n.* Stopping

Ocultación *n.* Masking; *n.* Supression

Odinofagia *n.* Odynophagia

Oído Externo *n.* Outer Ear

Oído Interno *n.* Inner Ear

Oído Medio *n.* Middle Ear

Olfato *n.* Olfaction

Oligodendrocito *n.* Oligodendrocyte

Omisión *n.* Omission

Omóplato *n.* Scapula; *n.* Shoulder Blade

Onda *n.* Wave

Onomatopeya *n.* Onomatopoeia

Oración *n.* Sentence; *n.* Oration

Organización Benéfico *n.* Charity

Organización Sin Fines de Lucro (OSFL) *n.* Nonprofit Organization

Órgano de Corti *n.* Organ of Corti; *n.* Spiral Organ

Orofacial *a.* Orofacial

Orofaringe *n.* Oropharynx

Orogástrico *a.* Orogastric

Oronasal *a.* Oronasal

Ortografía *n.* Orthography

Oscilación *n.* Oscillation

Óseo *a.* Osseus

Osteofito *n.* Osteophyte

Otitis Media (Aguda/ Crónica) *n.* Otitis Media (Acute/ Chronic)

Otolito *n.* Otolith

Otólogo *n.* Otologist

Otorrinolaringólogo *n.* ENT Specialist; *n.* Otorhinolaryngologist

Otoscopia *n.* Otoscopy

Otoscopio *n.* Otoscope; *n.* Auriscope

Ototóxico *a.* Ototoxic

Oyente *n.* Listener; *n.* Receiver

P

Pabellón Auricular *n.* Pinna; *n.* Auricle

Paciente *n.* Patient

Paladar *n.* Palate; *n.* Roof of the Mouth

Paladar Blando *n.* Soft Palate

Paladar Duro *n.* Hard Palate

Paladar Hendido *n.* Cleft Palate

Palatal *a.* Palatal

Palatalización *n.* Palatalization

Palatoalveolar *a.* Palatoalveolar

Palatofaríngeo *a.* Palatopharyngeal

Palatoplastia *n.* Palatoplasty

Palilalia *n.* Palilalia

Papeleo *n.* Paperwork

Papilas Circunvaladas *n.* Circumvallate Papillae

Papiloma *n.* Papilloma

Papilomatosis *n.* Papillomatosis

Par Craneal *n.* Cranial Nerve

Par Mínimo *n.* Minimal Pair

Parafasia *n.* Paraphasia

Paralelo *a.* Parallel

Parálisis *n.* Paralysis

Parálisis Bilateral de las Cuerdas Vocales *n.* Bilateral Vocal Cord Paralysis

Parálisis Bulbar *n.* Bulbar Palsy

Parálisis Cerebral *n.* Cerebral Palsy

Parálisis Pseudobulbar *n.* Pseudobulbar Paralysis

Parálisis Unilateral de las Cuerdas Vocales *n.* Unilateral Vocal Cord Paralysis

Parálisis de Bell *n.* Bell's Palsy

Paralizado *a.* Paralyzed

Paramédico *n.* Paramedic

Paranoia *n.* Paranoia

Paranoico *a.* Paranoid

Paraplejía *n.* Paraplegia

Paraprofesional *a.* Paraprofessional

Parental *a.* Parental

Paresia *n.* Paresis

Parte Opercular *n.* Opercular Part

Parte Triangular *n.* Triangular Part

Pascal *n.* Pascal

Patología *n.* Pathology

Patología del Habla y Lenguaje *n.* Speech-Language Pathology

Patológico *a.* Pathological

Patólogo *n.* Pathologist

Pausa *n.* Pause

Pecíolo Epiglótico *n.* Epiglottic Petiole

Pedagogía *n.* Pedagogy

Pedagógico *a.* Pedagogical

Pediátrico *a.* Pediatric

Penetración *n.* Penetration

Percepción Espacial *n.* Spatial Awareness

Percepción del Habla *n.* Speech Perception

Pérdida Auditiva *n.* Hearing Loss

Pérdida Auditiva Conductiva *n.* Conductive Hearing Loss

Pérdida Auditiva Inducida por Ruido *n.* Noise-Induced Hearing Loss

Pérdida Auditiva Mixta *n.* Mixed Hearing Loss

Pérdida Auditiva Sensorineural *n.* Sensorineural Hearing Loss

Pérdida de Memoria *n.* Memory Loss

Performativo *a.* Performative

Periférico *a.* Peripheral

Perilinfa *n.* Perilymph

Perinatal *a.* Perinatal

Periódico *a.* Periodic

Periodo de Atención *n.* Attention Span

Periodo Crítico *n.* Critical Period

Peristalsis *n.* Peristalsis

Permanencia de los Objetos n. Object Permanence

Perseverancia *n.* Perserverance

Pertinencia *n.* Relevance

Piamadre *n.* Pia Mater

Pidgin *n.* Pidgin

Pieza de Mordida *n.* Bite Block

Piramidal *a.* Pyramidal

Piriforme *a.* Pyriform

Pleura *n.* Pleura

Pliegue Vestibular *n.* Vestibular Fold

Pliegue Vocal *n.* Vocal Fold

Pliegues Ariepiglóticos *n.* Aryepiglottic Folds

Plurilingüe *a.* Multilingual

Poda Neuronal *n.* Synaptic Pruning

Políglota *n.* Polyglot

Pólipo *n.* Polyp

Política de Privacidad de HIPAA *n.* HIPAA Policy

Polo *n.* Pole

Porcentaje *n.* Percentage

Posgrado Clínico *n.* Clinical Fellowship

Posnatal *a.* Postnatal

Posprandial *a.* Postprandial; *a.* Postmeal

Post Mortem *a.* Post Mortem

Postalveolar *a.* Postalveolar

Posterior *a.* Posterior

Posteriorización *n.* Backing

Posteriorizado *a.* Backed

Postura *n.* Posture

Postural *a.* Postural

Potencial de Acción *n*. Action Potential

Potencial Eléctrico *n*. Electric Potential

Práctica Basada en la Evidencia (PBE) *n*. Evidence-Based Practice (EBP)

Pragmática *n*. Pragmatics

Prealfabetización *n*. Preliteracy

Precanceroso *a*. Precancerous

Precisión *n*. Precision

Predisposición *n*. Predisposition

Preescolar *a*. Preschool

Prefijo *n*. Prefix

Prejuicio *n*. Prejudice

Prelingüístico *a*. Prelinguistic

Prematuro *a*. Premature

Prepalatal *a*. Postalveolar;

Preparatoria *n*. High School

Presbiacusia *n*. Presbycusis; *n*. Presbyacusis

Presbiafagia *n.* Presbyphagia

Presbilaringe *n.* Presbylarynx; *n.* Presbylaryngis

Prescribir *v.* Prescribe

Prescriptivismo *n.* Prescriptivism; *n.* Prescriptive Grammar

Prescriptivista *n.* Prescriptivist; *a.* Prescriptive

Presión *n.* Pressure

Presión Alta *n.* High Blood Pressure; *n.* Hypertension

Presión de Aire *n.* Air Pressure

Presión Positiva Continua en la Vía Respiratoria (CPAP) *n.* Continuous Positive Airway Pressure (CPAP)

Presión Intracraneal (PIC) *n.* Intracranial Pressure (ICP)

Presonorización *n.* Prevoicing

Préstamo *n.* Loan Word

Prestigio *n.* Prestige

Pretérmino *a.* Preterm

Prevalencia *n.* Prevalence

Prevocálico *a.* Prevocalic

Primario *a.* Primary

Probabilidad *n.* Probability

Procedimiento *n.* Procedure

Procesamiento Auditivo Central *n.* Central Auditory Processing

Proceso Alveolar *n.* Alveolar Process

Procesos Fonológicos *n.p.* Phonological Processes

Profesor de Voz *n.* Voice Coach

Prognatismo *n.* Prognathism

Programación *n.* Scheduling

Programa de Educación Individualizado (IEP) *n.* Individualized Education Program (IEP)

Progresivo *a.* Progressive

Progreso *n.* Progress

Pronóstico *n.* Prognosis

Proporción *n.* Ratio; *n.* Proportion

Propósito *n*. Purpose; *n*. Aim; *n*. Objective

Propriocepción *n*. Proprioception

Prosencéfalo *n*. Prosencephalon; *n*. Forebrain

Prosodia *n*. Prosody

Prosódico *a*. Prosodic

Proteína *n*. Protein

Proteína Tau *n*. Tau Protein

Protésico *a*. Prosthetic

Protésis *n*. Prosthesis

Prótesis Palatal *n*. Palatal Lift; *n*. Palatal Prosthesis

Prototipo *n*. Prototype

Protruir *v*. Protrude

Protrusión *n*. Protrusion

Protuberancia Anular *n*. Pons

Proxémica *n*. Proxemics

Proximal *a*. Proximal

Prueba *n.* Test

Prueba de Cribado *n.* Screening Test

Prueba de la Falsa Creencia *n.* Sally-Anne Test

Prueba de Wada *n.* Wada Test

Pruebas de Laboratorio en el Lugar de Asistencia (POCT) *n.* Point-of-Care Testing (POCT)

Pruebas Referidas a Criterios *n.p.* Criterion-Referenced Tests

Pruebas Referidas a la Norma *n.p.* Norm-Referenced Tests

Pseudociencia *n.* Pseudoscience

Psicógeno *a.* Psychogenic

Psicolingüística *n.* Psycholinguistics

Psicología *n.* Psychology

Psicológico *a.* Psychological

Psicólogo *n.* Psychologist

Psicosis *n.* Psychosis

Psicosomático *a.* Psychosomatic

Psiquiatra *n.* Psychiatrist

Psiquiatría *n.* Psychiatry

Ptosis *n.* Ptosis

Pubertad *n.* Puberty

Pubis *n.* Pubis

Pudín *n.* Pudding

Puente de Varolio *n.* Pons

Puente Troncoencefálico *n.* Pons

Puerto Velofaríngeo *n.* Velopharyngeal Port; *n.* Velopharyngeal Sphincter

Pulmonar *a.* Pulmonary; *a.* Pulmonic

Pulmones *n.* Lungs

Punto de Articulación *n.* Place of Articulation; *n.* Point of Articulation

Puntuación de Apgar *n.* Apgar Score

Puré *n.* Puree

Putamen *n.* Putamen

Q

Queratosis *n.* Keratosis

Quiasma Óptico *n.* Optic Chiasm

Quimioterapia *n.* Chemotherapy

Quinesiología *n.* Kinesiology

Quinesiólogo *n.* Kinesiologist

Quirófano *n.* Operating Room (OR)

Quiste *n.* Cyst

R

Racismo *n.* Racism

Radiación *n.* Radiation

Radiografía *n.* X-Ray

Radiográfico *a.* Radiographic

Radioterapia *n.* Radiotherapy

Rafe *n.* Raphe

Rampa Coclear *n.* Scala Media; *n.* Cochlear Duct

Rampa Timpánica *n.* Scala Tympani; *n.* Tympanic Duct

Rampa Vestibular *n.* Scala Vestibuli; *n.* Vestibular Duct

Rango *n.* Range

Raro *a.* Rare

Rasgo Semántico *n.* Semantic Feature

Rayos X *n.* X-Rays

Reacción *n.* Reaction; *n.* Response

Real Academia Española (RAE) *n.* Royal Spanish Academy (RAE)

Reanimación *n.* Resuscitation

Reanimación Cardiopulmonar (RCP) *n.* Cardiopulmonary Resuscitation (CPR)

Receta *n.* Prescription

Recetar *v.* Prescribe

Reciprocidad *n.* Reciprocity

Reconocer *v.* Recognize

Reconocimiento *n.* Recognition

Reconocimiento del Habla *n.* Speech Recognition

Redondeado *a.* Rounded

Redondeamiento *n.* Rounding

Recuperación *n.* Recovery

Recurrente *n.* Recurring; *n.* Intermittent

Reducción *n.* Reduction

Reduplicación *n.* Reduplication

Referencia *n.* Reference

Referencial *a.* Referential

Reflejo *n.* Reflex

Reflejo de Babinski *n.* Babinski Reflex; *n.* Babinski Sign

Reflejo de Búsqueda *n.* Rooting Reflex

Reflejo de Succión *n.* Sucking Reflex

Reflejo Nauseoso *n.* Gag Reflex

Reflujo *n.* Reflux; *n.* Backflow

Reflujo Gástrico *n.* Gastric Reflux

Reflujo Laringofaríngeo *n.* Laryngopharyngeal Reflux

Reforzamiento *n.* Reinforcement

Reforzamiento Negativo *n.* Negative Reinforcement

Reforzamiento Positivo *n.* Positive Reinforcement

Registro *n.* Register

Registro Glotal *n.* Glottal Fry; *n.* Glottal Register; *n.* Vocal Fry

Regla *n.* Rule

Regresión *n.* Regression

Rehabilitación *n.* Rehabilitation

Rehabilitación Auditiva *n.* Aural Rehabilitation

Rehilamiento *n.* Assibilation

Relación Señal-Ruido (SNR) (S/R) *n.* Signal-Noise Ratio (SNR) (S/N)

Relación S/Z *n.* S/Z Ratio

Relevancia *n.* Relevance

Remisión *n.* Remission

Reparación *n.* Remediation

Repetición *n.* Repetition

Resección *n.* Resection

Resfriado Común *n.* Common Cold

Resguardado *a.* Sheltered

Residual *a.* Residual

Residuo *n.* Residue

Resistencia *n.* Resistance

Resolución de Problemas *n.* Problem Solving

Resonador *n.* Resonator

Resonancia *n.* Resonance

Resonancia Oral *n.* Oral Resonance

Respiración *n.* Respiration; *n.* Breathing

Respiración Glosofaríngea *n.* Glossopharyngeal Breathing; *n.* Frog Breathing

Respiración Silenciosa *n.* Quiet Breathing

Respuesta Auditiva del Tronco Encefálico (RATE) *n.* Auditory Brainstem Response (ABR)

Respuesta Física Total (TPR) *n.* Total Physical Response (TPR)

Resultado *n.* Result; *n.* Outcome

Retardado *a.* Delayed

Retracción *n.* Backing; *n.* Retraction

Retraído *a.* Backed; *a.* Retracted

Retrasado *a.* Delayed

Retraso *n.* Delay

Retraso de Desarrollo *n.* Developmental Delay; *n.* Developmental Gap

Retraso de Lenguaje *n.* Language Delay; *n.* Developmental Language Disorder (DLD)

Retroalimentación *n.* Feedback

Retrococlear *a.* Retrocochlear

Retrofleja *a.* Retroflex

Reversible *a.* Reversible

Revisado por Pares *a.* Peer-Reviewed

Revisión Anual *n.* Annual Review

Rima *n.* Rhyme

Ritmo *n.* Pace; *n.* Rate; *n.* Rhythm; *n.* Speed

Ritmo Estable *n.* Steady Rate; *n.* Steady Pace

Ritmo del Habla *n.* Rate of Speech

Rombencéfalo *n.* Hindbrain; *n.* Rhombencephalon

Ronquera *n.* Hoarseness

Rotacismo *n*. Rhotacism

Rótico *a*. Rhotic

S

Sacro *n.* Sacrum

Sagital *a.* Sagittal

Saliente *a.* Salient

Salino *a.* Saline

Saliva *n.* Saliva

Salival *a.* Salivary

Salón de Recursos *n.* Resource Room

Saturación *n.* Saturation

Schwanoma Vestibular *n.* Vestibular Schwannoma; *n.* Acoustic Neuroma

Script *n.* Script

Secreción *n.* Secretion

Secuencia *n.* Sequence

Secundario *a.* Secondary

Segmento *n.* Segment

Segmentación *n.* Segmentation

Segunda Lengua *n.* Second Language

Seis Sonidos de Ling *n.p.* Ling Six Sounds

Semántica *n.* Semantics; *a.* Semantic

Semiconsonante *n.* Semiconsonant

Semivocal *n.* Semivowel; *n.* Glide

Senil *a.* Senile

Seno *n.* Sinus

Sensación *n.* Sensation

Sensación de Globo *n.* Globus Sensation

Sensible *a.* Sensitive

Sensorial *a.* Sensory

Señal *n.* Cue; *n.* Signal

Señalización *n.* Signaling; *n.* Cueing

Serosa *n.* Serous Membrane

Servicios de Protección de Niños (CPS) *n.p.* Child Protective Services (CPS)

[283]

Sesgo *n*. Bias

Severo *a*. Severe

Sexismo *n*. Sexism

Shimmer *n*. Shimmer

Sibilante *n*. Sibilant ; *a*. Sibilant

Significado *n*. Meaning

Sílaba *n*. Syllable

Silabificación *n*. Syllabification

Símbolo Diacrítico *n*. Diacritic

Símbolos Bliss *n.p*. Blissymbols

Simplificación *n*. Simplification

Sinalefa *n*. Synalepha

Sinapsis *n*. Synapse

Sináptico *a*. Synaptic

Sinaptogénesis *n*. Synaptogenesis

Síndrome *n*. Syndrome

Síndrome Alcohólico Fetal (SAF) *n.* Fetal Alcohol Syndrome (FAS)

Síndrome Cardiofaciocutáneo (CFC) *n.* Cardiofaciocutaneous Syndrome (CFC)

Síndrome CHARGE *n.* CHARGE Syndrome

Síndrome de Asperger (AS) *n.* Asperger Syndrome (AS)

Síndrome de Dehiscencia del Canal Superior (SCDS) *n.* Superior Canal Dehiscence Syndrome (SCDS)

Síndrome de Down *n.* Down Syndrome

Síndrome de Guillain-Barré (GBS) *n.* Guillain-Barré Syndrome (GBS)

Síndrome de Inmunodeficiencia Adquirida (SIDA) *n.* Acquired Immunodeficiency Syndrome (AIDS)

Síndrome del Cromosoma X Frágil (SFX) *n.* Fragile X Syndrome (FXS)

Síndrome del Hemisferio Derecho (RHD) *n.* Right Hemisphere Disorder (RHD)

Síndrome de Muerte Súbita del Lactante (SMSL) *n.* Sudden Infant Death Syndrome (SIDS)

Síndrome de Pfeiffer *n*. Pfeiffer Syndrome

Síndrome de Tourette (TS) *n*. Tourette Syndrome (TS)

Síndrome Velocardiofacial (VCFS) *n*. Velocardiofacial Syndrome (VCFS)

Síndrome de Williams (WS) *n*. Williams Syndrome (WS)

Síndrome Disejecutivo (SD) *n*. Dysexecutive Syndrome (DES)

Síndrome Talámico *n*. Thalamic Pain Syndrome; *n*. Dejerine–Roussy Syndrome

Sínfisis *n*. Symphysis

Singulto *n*. Singultus

Sintaxis *n*. Syntax

Síntesis *n*. Synthesis

Síntoma *n*. Symptom

Síntoma de Babinski *n*. Babinski's Sign ; *n*. Babinski's Reflex

Sinusoidal *a*. Sinusoid

Sinusoide *n*. Sinusoid

Sistema Digestivo *n*. Digestive System; *n*. Digestive Tract

Sistema Límbico *n*. Limbic System

Sistema Nervioso *n*. Nervous System

Sistema Nervioso Autónomo *n*. Autonomic Nervous System

Sistema Nervioso Central (SNC) *n*. Central Nervous System (CNS)

Sistema Nervioso Periférico (SNP) *n*. Peripheral Nervous System (PNS)

Sistema Nervioso Simpático *n*. Sympathetic Nervous System

Sistema de Comunicación por Intercambio de Imágenes (PECS) *n*. Picture Exchange Communication System (PECS)

Sobremordida *n*. Overbite

Sociolingüística *n*. Sociolinguistics

Sonante *n*. Sonorant; *n*. Resonant

Sonda *n*. Tube; *n*. Probe

Sonda Gástrica *n*. Gavage; *n*. Gastric Tube

Sonido *n.* Sound

Sonoridad *n.* Sonority; Voicing

Sonoro *a.* Voiced

Soplo *n.* Bruit; *n.* Murmur

Sordera *n.* Deafness

Sordera Cortical *n.* Cortical Deafness

Sordera Verbal *n.* Pure Word Deafness; *n.* Auditory Verbal Agnosia (AVA)

Sordo *a.* Deaf

Subagudo *a.* Subacute

Subaracnoideo *a.* Subarachnoid

Subdural *a.* Subdural

Subglótico *a.* Subglottal

Subtálamo *n.* Subthalamus

Sucesivo *a.* Successive

Sufijo *n.* Suffix

Superficial *a.* Superficial

Superior *a.* Superior; *a.* Upper

Suplementación del Alfabeto *n.* Alphabet Supplementation

Suplemento Dietético *n.* Dietary Supplement

Supracricoideo *a.* Supracricoid

Supraglótico *a.* Supraglottal

Supraoclusión *n.* Overbite

Supresión *n.* Deletion

Supresión de Consonantes Finales *n.* Final Consonant Deletion

Supresión de Consonantes Iniciales *n.* Initial Consonant Deletion

Supresión de Consonantes Mediales *n.* Medial Consonant Deletion

Supresión de Sílabas Átonas *n.* Weak Syllable Deletion

Surco *n.* Sulcus

Surco Calcarino *n.* Calcarine Sulcus

Surco Central *n.* Central Sulcus; *n.* Fissure of Rolando

Surco Lateral *n.* Lateral Sulcus; *n.* Sylvian Fissure

Sustancia Blanca *n.* White Matter

Sustancia Gris *n.* Gray Matter

Sustancia Negra *n.* Substantia Nigra

Sustitución *n.* Substitution

Sustituir *v.* Substitute

Sutura *n.* Suture

T

Táctil *a.* Tactile

Talámico *a.* Thalamic

Tálamo *n.* Thalamus

Talla Media de la Expresión (MLU) *n.* Mean Length of Utterance (MLU)

Tallo Epiglótico *n.* Epiglottic Petiole

Tanteo *n.* Groping

Taquicardia *n.* Tachycardia

Tartamudear *v.* Stutter

Tartamudez *n.* Stuttering

Tasa Diadococinética *n.* Diadochokinetic Rate (DDK)

Tejido *n.* Tissue

Telencéfalo *n.* Telencephalon; *n.* Endbrain

Telepráctica *n.* Telepractice

Teleterapia *n.* Teletherapy

Temblor *n.* Tremor

Temblor de Reposo *n.* Rest Tremor

Temblor Esencial (TE) *n.* Essential Tremor (ET)

Temblor Intencional *n.* Intention Tremor

Temblor Vocal *n.* Vocal Tremor; *n.* Organic Voice Tremor

Tensión *n.* Tensión; *n.* Voltage

Tensión Vocal *n.* Vocal Tension

Teoría *n.* Theory

Teoría de la Mente *n.* Theory of Mind

Teoría del Desarrollo Cognitivo de Piaget *n.* Piaget's Theory of Cognitive Development

Teoría Hebbiana *n.* Hebbian Theory

Terapeuta Ocupacional *n.* Occupational Therapist

Terapeuta de la Alimentación *n.* Feeding Therapist

Terapia *n.* Therapy

Terapia Ambiental *n.* Milieu Therapy

Terapia Auditivo-Verbal (TAV) *n.* Auditory-Verbal Therapy (AVT)

Terapia de Entonación Melódica (TEM) *n.* Melodic Intonation Therapy (MIT)

Terapia Familiar *n.* Family Therapy

Terapia Intensiva *n.* Intensive Therapy

Terapia Ocupacional *n.* Occupational Therapy

Terapia Recreativa *n.* Recreational Therapy

Terapia de Juego *n.* Play Therapy

Terapia del Habla *n.* Speech Therapy

Terapia del Viaje *n.* Travel Therapy

Teratogénesis *n.* Teratogenesis

Tic *n.* Tic

Tilde *n.* Accent Mark

Tímpano *n.* Eardrum; *n.* Tympanic Membrane

Timpanometría *n.* Tympanometry

Tinnitus *n.* Tinnitus

Tipo *n.* Type

Tiroides *n.* Thyroid

Tiroplastia *n.* Thyroplasty

Tomar Turnos *v.* Turn Taking

Tomografía Computarizada (TC) *n.* Computed Tomography (CT); *n.* Computed Axial Tomography (CAT)

Tomografía por Emisión de Positrones (TEP) *n.* Positron Emission Tomography (PET)

Tónico *a.* Stressed

Tono *n.* Pitch; *n.* Tone

Tono Muscular *n.* Muscle Tone

Tonotópico *a.* Tonotopic

Tonsilitis *n.* Tonsillitis

Torácico *n.* Thyroid

Tortícolis *n.* Torticollis

Tos *n.* Cough

Toxina Botulínica (Bótox) *n.* Botulinum Toxin (Botox)

Tracto *n.* Tract

Tracto Corticobulbar *n.* Corticobulbar Tract

Tracto Corticoespinal *n.* Corticospinal Tract

Tracto Vocal *n.* Vocal Tract

Traducción *n.* Translation

Traducir *v.* Translate

Trámites *n.* Paperwork

Transcripción *n.* Transcription

Transcripción Amplia *n.* Broad Transcription

Transcripción Detallada *n.* Narrow Transcription

Transcripción Fonémica *n.* Phonemic Transcription

Transcripción Fonética *n.* Phonetic Transcription

Transgénero *a.* Transgender

Transglótico *a.* Transglottal

Transitorio *a.* Transient; *a.* Transitional

Transversal *a.* Transverse

Trapecio *n.* Trapezius

Tráquea *n.* Trachea

Traqueoesofágico *a.* Tracheoesophageal

Traqueomalacia *n.* Tracheomalacia

Traqueostomía *n.* Tracheostomy

Traqueotomía *n.* Tracheotomy

Traspaso *n.* Carryover; *n.* Crossing over; *n.* Transfer

Trastorno Adquirido del Habla *n.* Acquired Speech Disorder

Trastorno Bipolar *n.* Bipolar Disorder

Trastorno Cromosómico *n.* Chromosomal Disorder

Trastorno de Omisión *n.* Hemispatial Neglect

Trastorno del Desarrollo del Lenguaje (TDL) *n.* Developmental Language Disorder (DLD)

Trastorno Específico del Lenguaje (TEL) *n.* Developmental Language Disorder (DLD); *n.* Specific Language Impairment (SLI)

Trastorno Límite de la Personalidad (TLP) *n.* Borderline Personality Disorder (BPD)

Trastorno Motor del Habla *n.* Motor Speech Disorder

Trastorno Orgánico *n.* Organic Disorder

Trastorno de Ansiedad Generalizada (TAG) *n.* Generalized Anxiety Disorder (GAD)

Trastorno de Deglución *n.* Swallowing Disorder

Trastorno de Lenguaje *n.* Language Disorder; *n.* Developmental Language Disorder (DLD)

Trastorno de Personalidad *n.* Personality Disorder

Trastorno de Procesamiento Auditivo Central (TPAC) *n.* Central Auditory Processing Disorder (CAPD)

Trastorno de Voz *n.* Voice Disorder

Trastorno del Habla *n.* Speech Disorder

Trastorno Miofuncional Orofacial (OMD) *n.* Orofacial Myofunctional Disorder (OMD)

Trastorno por Déficit de Atención con Hiperactividad (TDAH) *n.* Attention Deficit Hyperactivity Disorder (ADHD)

Trastornos de la Comunicación *n.* Communication Disorders

Trastorno del Espectro del Autismo (TEA) *n.* Autism Spectrum Disorder (ASD)

Tratamiento *n.* Treatment; *n.* Therapy

Tratamiento de la Deglución *n.* Swallowing Therapy; *n.* Swallowing Treatment

Trauma *n.* Trauma

Traumático *a.* Traumatic

Traumatismo *n.* Injury; *n.* Trauma; *n.* Lesion

Tremulante *n.* Rhotic

Triaje *n.* Triage

Trígrafo *n.* Trigraph

Trilingüe *a.* Trilingual

Triptongo *n.* Triphthong

Trisomía *n.* Trisomy

Trombectomía *n.* Thrombectomy

Trombo *n.* Thrombus

Trombosis *n.* Thrombosis

Trompa de Eustaquio *n.* Eustachian Tube; *n.* Pharyngotympanic Tube; *n.* Auditory Tube

Tronco Encefálico *n.* Brainstem

Tubo Faringotimpánico *n.* Pharyngotympanic Tube; *n.* Eustachian Tube; *n.* Auditory Tube

Tubo Laríngeo *n.* Laryngeal Tube

Tubo Neural *n.* Neural Tube

Tumor *n.* Tumor

U

Úlcera *n.* Ulcer

Ultrasonido *n.* Ultrasound

Umbral *n.* Threshold

Unidad de Cuidados Intensivos (UCI) *n.* Intensive Care Unit (ICU)

Unidad de Cuidados Intensivos Neonatales (UCIN) *n.* Neonatal Intensive Care Unit (NICU)

Unidad de Educación Continua (CEU) *n.* Continuing Education Unit (CEU)

Unilateral *a.* Unilateral

Unión *n.* Union; *n.* Joining; *n.* Coalescence

Unión Mioneural *n.* Myoneural Junction

Unión Neuromuscular *n.* Neuromuscular Junction

Universidad *n.* University

Úvula *n.* Uvula

Uvular *a.* Uvular

V

Vacuna *n*. Vaccine

Vacunación *n*. Vaccination

Vagotomía *n*. Vagotomy

Vaina de Mielina *n*. Myelin Sheath

Validez *n*. Validity

Vallécula *n*. Vallecula

Valor Medio *n*. Mean Value

Válvula *n*. Valve

Variabilidad *n*. Variability

Variable *n*. Variable

Vascular *a*. Vascular

Vasovagal *a*. Vasovagal

Velar *a*. Velar

Velarización *n*. Velarization

Velo *n*. Soft Palate; *n*. Velum

Velocidad *n.* Speed; *n.* Rate

Velofaríngeo *a.* Velopharyngeal

Vena *n.* Vein

Ventana Oval *n.* Oval Window

Ventana Redonda *n.* Round Window

Ventral *a.* Ventral

Ventricular *a.* Ventricular

Ventrículo *n.* Ventricle

Verbal *a.* Verbal

Vernáculo *n.* Vernacular

Vértebra *n.* Vertebra

Vértigo *n.* Vertigo

Vestíbulo *n.* Vestibule

Veterano *n.* Veteran

Vía *n.* Pathway

Vía Aérea con Mascarilla Laríngea (VAML) *n.* Laryngeal Mask Airway (LMA)

Vías Respiratorias *n.p.* Airways; *n.p.* Respiratory Passages; *n.* Respiratory Tract

Vibración *n.* Vibration

Vibrante Múltiple *n.* Trill

Vibrante Simple *n.* Tap; *n.* Flap

Vibrar *v.* Vibrate

Video Fluoroscópico *a.* Videofluoroscopic

Viejismo *n.* Ageism

Virus de la Inmunodeficiencia Humana (VIH) *n.* Human Immunodeficiency Virus (HIV)

Visceral *a.* Visceral

Viscosidad *n.* Viscosity

Viscoso *a.* Viscous

Viseme *n.* Viseme

Visita en Domicilio *n.* House Call

Visomotriz *a.* Visual Motor

Vocabulario *n.* Vocabulary

Vocabulario Núcleo *n.* Core Vocabulary

Vocal *n.* Vowel

Vocal Abierta *n.* Open Vowel; *n.* Low Vowel

Vocal Alta *n.* High Vowel; *n.* Close Vowel

Vocal Anterior *n.* Front Vowel

Vocal Baja *n.* Low Vowel; *n.* Open Vowel

Vocal Casiabierta *n.* Near-Open Vowel; *n.* Near-Low Vowel

Vocal Casicerrada *n.* Near-Close Vowel; *n.* Near-High Vowel

Vocal Central *n.* Central Vowel

Vocal Cerrada *n.* Close Vowel; *n.* High Vowel

Vocal Corta *n.* Short Vowel

Vocal Intermedia *n.* Mid Vowel

Vocal Larga *n.* *n.* Long Vowel

Vocal Laxa *n.* Lax Vowel

Vocal Posterior *n.* Back Vowel

Vocal Semiabierta *n.* Open-Mid Vowel; *n.* Low-Mid Vowel

Vocal Semianterior *n.* Near-Front Vowel

Vocal Semicerrada *n.* Close-Mid Vowel; *n.* High-Mid Vowel

Vocal Semiposterior *n.* Near-Back Vowel

Vocal Tensa *n.* Tense Vowel

Vocalización *n.* Vocalization

Vocoide *n.* Vocoid

Volante (de) *n.* Referral (from)

Volitivo *a.* Volitional

Volumen *n.* Volume

Volumen del Conducto Auditivo Externo (ECV) *n.* Ear Canal Volume (ECV)

Voluntario *a.* Voluntary; *n.* Volunteer

Voz *n.* Voice

Voz Entrecortada *n.* Breathy Voice; *n.* Faltering Voice; *n.* Cracking Voice

(de) Voz Suave *a*. Softspoken

Y

Yunque *n.* Incus

Z

Zona de Desarrollo Próximo (ZDP) *n.* Zone of Proximal
Development (ZPD)

Appendix I: Tables and Figures

Place/Lugar		Manner/Manera	
Bilabial	Bilabial	Stop/Plosive	Oclusiva
Labiodental	Labiodental	Nasal	Nasal
Interdental	Interdental	Trill	Vibrante Múltiple
Alveolar/Postalveolar	Alveolar/Postalveolar	Flap/Tap	Vibrante Simple
Retroflex	Retrofleja	Fricative	Fricativa
Palatal	Palatal	Approximant	Aproximante
Velar	Velar	Glide	Deslizada
Uvular	Uvular	Liquid	Líquido
Pharyngeal	Faríngea	Lateral	Lateral
Glottal	Glotal	Rhotic	Rótica

Figure 1: Describing Place and Manner of Consonants

[310]

Voicing	
Voiced	Sonora
Voiceless	Insonora/Sorda

Figure 2: Describing Voicing of Consonant Sounds

Close/High	Cerrada/Alta
Mid	Intermedia
Open/Low	Abierta/Baja
Front	Anterior
Central	Central
Back	Posterior
Tense	Tensa
Lax	Laxa
Short	Corta
Long	Larga

Figure 3: Describing Vowel Sounds

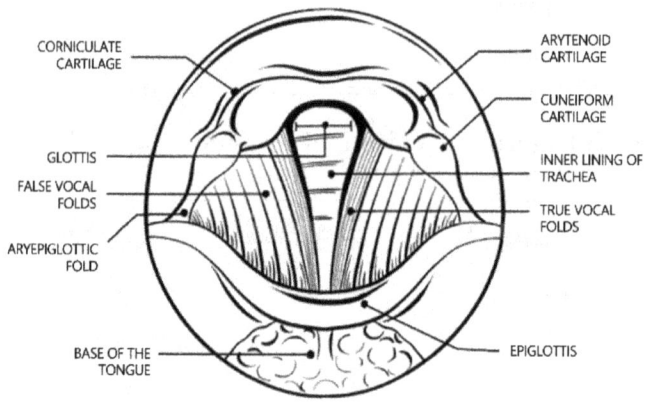

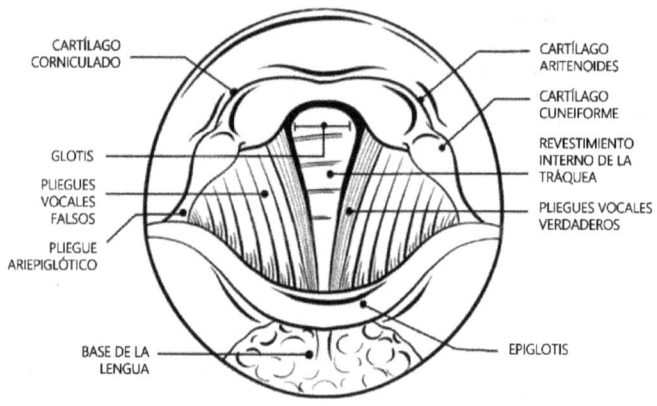

Figure 4: "Superior View of the Larynx, English and Spanish" Copyright © 2023 Devin Lukachik

Initial/Medial/Final Consonant Deletion	Omisión de Consonantes Iniciales/Medias/Finales	Voicing	Sonorización
Weak Syllable Deletion	Supresión de Sílabas Átonas	Reduplication	Reduplicación
Diphthong Deletion	Omisión de Diptongos	Lateralization	Lateralización
Nasalization	Nasalización	Epenthesis	Epéntesis
Backing	Posteriorización	Assimilation	Asimilación
Fronting	Anteriorización	Cluster Reduction	Reducción de Grupos Consonánticos
Gliding	Deslización	Metathesis	Metátesis
Devoicing	Desonorización	Stopping	Oclusivización

Figure 5: Selected Phonological Processes

[313]

I	Olfactory	Olfatorio
II	Optic	Óptico
III	Oculomotor	Óculomotor
IV	Trochlear	Troclear
V	Trigeminal	Trigémino
VI	Abducens	Abducens/Motor Ocular Externo
VII	Facial	Facial
VIII	Auditory/Vestibulocochlear	Auditivo/Vestibulococlear
IX	Glossopharyngeal	Glosofaríngeo
X	Vagus	Vago
XI	Accessory	Accesorio/Espinal
XII	Hypoglossal	Hipogloso

Figure 6: Cranial Nerves

[314]

Appendix II: Selected Abbreviations in English

AA *Anterograde Amnesia*

AAC *Augmentative and Alternative Communication*

AAVE *African-American Vernacular English*

ABA *Applied Behavior Analysis*

ABG *Arterial Blood Gas*

ABI *Acquired Brain Injury; Auditory Brainstem Implant*

ABR *Auditory Brainstem Response*

a.c. *Before Meals*

ACA *Anterior Cerebral Artery*

ADA *Americans with Disabilities Act; American Diabetes Association*

ADHD *Attention-Deficit/Hyperactivity Disorder*

ADL *Activity of Daily Living*

AIDS *Acquired Immunodeficiency Syndrome*

ALS *Amyotrophic Lateral Sclerosis*

AMA *Against Medical Advice*

AOS *Apraxia of Speech*

A/P *Anterior/Posterior*

ASD *Autism Spectrum Disorder*

ASHA *American Speech-Language-Hearing Association*

ASL *American Sign Language*

AVM *Arteriovenous Malformation*

AVT *Auditory-Verbal Therapy*

BAHA *Bone-Anchored Hearing Aid*

BBB *Blood-Brain Barrier*

BCBA *Board-Certified Behavior Analyst*

BG *Blood Glucose; Basal Ganglia*

BOT *Base of Tongue*

BP *Blood Pressure*

BPD *Borderline Personality Disorder*

BTE *Behind the Ear*

CA *Cardiac Arrest*

CAPD *Central Auditory Processing Disorder*

CAS *Childhood Apraxia of Speech*

CC *Chief Complaint; Cubic Centimeter*

CCC *Certificate of Clinical Competence*

CDC *Centers for Disease Control and Prevention*

CEA *Carotid Endarterectomy*

CEU *Continuing Education Unit*

CFC *Cardiofaciocutaneous Syndrome*

CHI *Closed Head Injury*

CIC *Completely in the Canal*

CN *Cranial Nerve*

CNA *Certified Nursing Assistant*

CNS *Central Nervous System*

COPD *Chronic Obstructive Pulmonary Disease*

COTA *Certified Occupational Therapy Assistant*

CP *Cerebral Palsy*

CPAP *Continuous Positive Airway Pressure*

CPR *Cardiopulmonary Resuscitation*

CPS *Child Protective Services*

CSF *Cerebrospinal Fluid*

CT *Computed Tomography*

CTE *Chronic Traumatic Encephalopathy*

CVA *Cerebrovascular Accident*

CXR *Chest X-Ray*

dB *Decibel*

DBS *Deep Brain Stimulation*

DC *Discharge*

DES *Dysexecutive Syndrome*

DHHS *Department of Health and Human Services*

DLD *Developmental Language Disorder*

DNA *Deoxyribonucleic Acid*

DNR *Do Not Resuscitate*

DNT *Did Not Test*

DOA *Dead on Arrival*

DOB *Date of Birth*

EAM *External Auditory Meatus*

EBP *Evidence-Based Practice*

ECoG *Electrocochleography*

ECV *Ear Canal Volume*

ED *Emergency Department*

EEG *Electroencephalography*

EF *Executive Function*

EFL *English as a Foreign Language*

EGG *Electroglottography*

EMT *Emergency Medical Technician; Enhanced Milieu Teaching*

ENT *Ear, Nose and Throat (Otorhinolaryngology)*

ESL *English as a Second Language*

ET *Essential Tremor*

FAS *Fetal Alcohol Syndrome*

FDA *Food and Drug Administration*

FEES *Fiberoptic Endoscopic Evaluation of Swallowing*

FEESST *Fiberoptic Endoscopic Evaluation of Swallowing with Sensory Testing*

FH *Family History*

fMRI *Functional Magnetic Resonance Imaging*

FTD *Frontotemporal Dementia*

FTLD *Frontotemporal Lobar Degeneration*

FXS *Fragile X Syndrome*

GABA *γ-Aminobutyric Acid*

GAD *Generalized Anxiety Disorder*

GBS *Guillain-Barré Syndrome*

GCS *Glasgow Coma Scale*

GE *Gastroenterology*

GERD *Gastroesophageal Reflux Disease*

GSW *Gunshot Wound*

HBP *High Blood Pressure*

HD *Huntington's Disease*

HIPAA *Health Insurance Portability and Accountability Act*

HL *Hearing Loss*

HNC *Head and Neck Cancer*

HPE *Holoprosencephaly*

HR *Heart Rate*

HTN *Hypertension*

Hz *Hertz*

ICP *Intracranial Pressure*

ID *Intellectual Disability*

IDEA *Individuals with Disabilities Education Act*

IEP *Individualized Education Program*

IPA *International Phonetic Alphabet*

IRB *Institutional Review Board*

ITE *In the Ear*

LBD *Lewy Body Dementia*

LD *Learning Disability*

LEP *Limited English Proficiency*

LES *Lower Esophageal Sphincter*

LGB *Lateral Geniculate Body*

LLE *Late Language Emergence*

LMA *Laryngeal Mask Airway*

LMN *Lower Motor Neuron*

LTM *Long-Term Memory*

MBSS *Modified Barium Swallow Study*

MCA *Middle Cerebral Artery*

MCI *Mild Cognitive Impairment*

MD *Doctor of Medicine; Muscular Dystrophy; Ménière's Disease*

MG *Myasthenia Gravis*

MGB *Medial Geniculate Body*

MI *Myocardial Infarction*

MIT *Melodic Intonation Therapy*

MLU *Mean Length of Utterance*

MRI *Magnetic Resonance Imaging*

MS *Multiple Sclerosis*

MVA *Motor Vehicle Accident*

NDD *National Dysphagia Diet*

NG *Nasogastric*

NICU *Neonatal Intensive Care Unit*

NPH *Normal Pressure Hydrocephalus*

NPO *Nil per os/Nothing by Mouth; Nonprofit Organization*

NTD *Neural Tube Defect*

OAE *Otoacoustic Emission*

OHI *Open Head Injury*

OM *Otitis Media*

OME *Otitis Media with Effusion*

OPCA *Olivopontocerebellar Atrophy*

OR *Operating Room*

PA *Physician's Assistant*

PAS *Penetration-Aspiration Scale*

PBA *Pseudobulbar Affect*

p.c. *After Meals*

PCA *Posterior Cerebral Artery*

PD *Parkinson's Disease*

PE *Pulmonary Embolism*

PECS *Picture Exchange Communication System*

PET *Positron Emission Tomography*

PEG *Percutaneous Endoscopic Gastrostomy*

PFC *Prefrontal Cortex*

PES *Pharyngoesophageal Segment*

POCT *Point-of-Care Testing*

PPA *Primary Progressive Aphasia*

PPAOS *Primary Progressive Apraxia of Speech*

PPF *Posterior Pharyngeal Flap*

RA *Retrograde Amnesia*

RHD *Right Hemisphere Disorder*

RIC *Receiver in Canal*

RLN *Recurrent Laryngeal Nerve*

RN *Registered Nurse*

SAH *Subarachnoid Hemorrhage*

SCDS *Superior Canal Dehiscence Syndrome*

SCI *Spinal Cord Injury*

SD *Spasmodic Dysphonia*

SDH *Subdural Hematoma*

SIDS *Sudden Infant Death Syndrome*

SLI *Specific Language Impairment*

SLN *Superior Laryngeal Nerve*

SLP *Speech-Language Pathologist*

SLPA *Speech-Language Pathology Assistant*

SM *Selective Mutism*

SNF *Skilled Nursing Facility*

SNR *Signal-to-Noise Ratio*

SOB *Shortness of Breath*

SOC *Superior Olivary Complex*

s/s *Signs and Symptoms*

STD *Sexually Transmitted Disease*

STI *Sexually Transmitted Infection*

STM *Short-Term Memory*

TBI *Traumatic Brain Injury*

TC *Total Communication*

TD *Tardive Dyskinesia*

TIA *Transient Ischemic Attack*

tPa *Tissue Plasminogen Activator*

TPN *Total Parenteral Nutrition*

TS *Tourette Syndrome*

UES *Upper Esophageal Sphincter*

UMN *Upper Motor Neuron*

URI *Upper Respiratory Infection*

VBI *Vertebrobasilar Insufficiency*

VCFS *Velocardiofacial Syndrome*

VF *Vocal Fold*

VFP *Vocal Fold Paralysis*

VPD *Velopharyngeal Dysfunction*

VPI *Velopharyngeal Insufficiency*

VPP *Velopharyngeal Port*

VWFA *Visual Word Form Area*

WNL *Within Normal Limits*

ZPD *Zone of Proximal Development*

Appendix III: Abreviaturas Seleccionadas en Español

AA *Amnesia Anterógrada*

ABA *Análisis del Comportamiento Aplicado*

a.c. *Antes de Comer*

ACA *Arteria Cerebral Anterior*

ACM *Arteria Cerebral Media*

ACP *Arteria Cerebral Posterior*

ACV *Accidente Cerebrovascular*

ACVD *Actividades de la Vida Diaria*

ADN *Ácido Desoxirribonucleico*

AFI *Alfabeto Fonético Internacional*

AIT *Ataque Isquémico Transitorio*

AOS *Apraxia del Habla*

A/P *Anterior/Posterior*

APP *Afasia Progresiva Primaria*

AR *Amnesia Retrógrada*

ASL *Lengua de Signos Americana*

AVM *Accidente de Vehículo de Motor*

BAHA *Audífono con Anclaje Óseo*

BHE *Barrera Hematoencefálica*

BTE *Retroauricular*

CAA *Comunicación Aumentativa y Alternativa*

CAE *Conducto Auditivo Externo*

CAS *Apraxia del Habla Infantil*

CCC *Certificado de Competencia Clínica*

CDC *Centros Para el Control y la Prevención de Enfermedades*

CIC *Completamente en el Canal*

COS *Complejo Olivar Superior*

CPAP *Presión Positiva Continua en la Vía Respiratoria*

CPS *Servicios de Protección de Niños*

dB *Decibelio*

DBS *Estimulación Cerebral Profunda*

DCL *Deterioro Cognitivo Leve*

DFT *Demencia Frontotemporal*

DLFT *Degeneración Lobular Frontotemporal*

DLN *Dentro de Límites Normales*

DND *Dieta Nacional de Disfagia*

DNR *No Resucitar*

DTA *Demencia Tipo Alzheimer*

DTN *Defecto del Tubo Neural*

EAC *Endarterectomía Carotídea*

EAI *Enfermedad Autoinmune*

ECoG *Electrococleografía*

ED *Evaluación Dinámica*

EEG *Electroencefalografía*

EEI *Esfínter Esofágico Inferior*

EES *Esfínter Esofágico Superior*

ELA *Esclerosis Lateral Amiotrófica*

EOA *Emisión Otoacústica*

EP *Embolia Pulmonar*

EPOC *Enfermedad Pulmonar Obstructiva Crónica*

ERGE *Enfermedad por Reflujo Gastroesofágico*

ESL *Inglés como Segunda Lengua*

ETC *Encefalopatía Traumática Crónica*

ETS *Enfermedad de Transmisión Sexual*

FEES *Evaluación Endoscópica de la Deglución por Fibra Óptica*

GBS *Síndrome de Guillain-Barré*

GEP *Gastrostomía Endoscópica Percutánea*

HIV *Human Immunodeficiency Virus*

HNT *Hidrocefalia Normotensiva*

HPE *Holoprosencefalia*

HSA *Hemorragia Subaracnoidea*

HSD *Hematoma Subdural*

HTN *Hipertensión*

IAM *Infarto Agudo de Miocardio*

IATC *Implante Auditivo de Tronco Cerebral*

IAV *Inglés Afroestadounidense Vernáculo*

IEP *Programa de Educación Individualizado*

IRM *Imagen por Resonancia Magnética*

IRMf *Imagen por Resonancia Magnética Funcional*

ITE *Intrauricular*

ITS *Infección de Transmisión Sexual*

IVB *Insuficiencia Vertebrobasilar*

LCA *Lesión Cerebral Adquirida*

LCE *Líquido Cerebroespinal*

LCT *Lesión Cerebral Traumática*

LEP *Dominio Limitado del Inglés*

LME *Lesión de la Médula Espinal*

LPC *La Palabra Complementada*

MAV *Malformación Arteriovenosa*

MBSS *Esofagografía con Bario*

MCP *Memoria a Corto Plazo*

MG *Miastenia Grave*

MLP *Memoria a Largo Plazo*

MLU *Talla Media de la Expresión*

MNI *Motoneurona Inferior*

MNS *Motoneurona Superior*

MV *Mecanismo Velofaríngeo*

NG *Nasogástrico*

NLR *Nervio Laríngeo Recurrente*

NLS *Nervio Laríngeo Superior*

NPO *Nil per os/ Nada por Vía Oral*

NPT *Nutrición Parenteral Total*

OM *Otitis Media*

OME *Otitis Media con Efusión*

ORL *Otorrinolaringología*

PAS *Escala de Penetración-Aspiración*

PBE *Práctica Basada en Evidencia*

p.c. *Después de Comer*

PC *Par Craneal*

PCV *Parálisis de Cuerdas Vocales*

PECS *Sistema de Comunicación por Intercambio de Imágenes*

PFC *Corteza Prefrontal*

PIC *Presión Intracraneal*

PPAOS *Apraxia Progresiva Primaria del Habla*

QTP *Quimioterapia*

RAE *Real Academia Española*

RATE *Respuesta Auditiva del Tronco Encefálico*

RCP *Reanimación Cardiopulmonar*

RIC *Receptor en el Canal*

RN *Recién Nacido*

RNpre *Recién Nacido Pretérmino*

RNpos *Recién Nacido Postérmino*

SAF *Síndrome Alcohólico Fetal*

SCDS *Síndrome de Dehiscencia del Canal Superior*

SD *Disfonía Espasmódica; Síndrome Disejecutivo*

SFX *Síndrome del Cromosoma X Frágil*

SIDA *Síndrome de Inmunodeficiencia Adquirida*

SM *Mutismo Selectivo*

SMSL *Síndrome de Muerte Súbita del Lactante*

SNC *Sistema Nervioso Central*

[333]

SNF *Centro de Enfermería Diestro*

SNP *Sistema Nervioso Periférico*

TAG *Trastorno de Ansiedad Generalizada*

TAV *Terapia Auditivo-Verbal*

TC *Tomografía Computarizada*

TDAH *Trastorno por Déficit de Atención con Hiperactividad*

TDL *Trastorno del Desarrollo del Lenguaje*

TE *Temblor Esencial*

TEA *Trastorno del Espectro del Autismo*

TEL *Trastorno Específico del Lenguaje*

TEM *Terapia de Entonación Melódica*

TEP *Tomografía por Emisión de Positrones*

TLP *Trastorno Límite de la Personalidad*

TPAC *Trastorno del Procesamiento Auditivo Central*

TRS *Tracto Respiratorio Superior*

TS *Síndrome de Tourette*

UCI *Unidad de Cuidados Intensivos*

UCIN *Unidad de Cuidados Intensivos Neonatales*

VAML *Vía Aérea con Mascarilla Laríngea*

VIH *Virus de la Inmunodeficiencia Humana*

ZDP *Zona de Desarrollo Próximo*

www.ingramcontent.com/pod-product-compliance
Lightning Source LLC
Chambersburg PA
CBHW072110270326
41931CB00010B/1512